Minding the Child

Minding the Child considers the implications of the concept of mentalization for a range of therapeutic interventions with children and families. Mentalization, and the empirical research which has supported it, now plays a significant role in a range of psychotherapies for adults. In this book we see how these rich ideas about the development of the self and interpersonal relatedness can help to foster the emotional well-being of children and young people in clinical practice and a range of other settings.

With contributions from a range of international experts, the three main parts of the book explore:

- the concept of mentalization from a theoretical and research perspective
- the value of mentalization-based interventions within child mental health services
- the application of mentalizing ideas to work in community settings.

Minding the Child will not only be of particular interest to clinicians and those working therapeutically with children and families, but will also be of interest to academics and students concerned with child and adolescent mental health, developmental psychology and the study of social cognition.

Nick Midgley is a Child and Adolescent Psychotherapist and Senior Research Fellow at the Anna Freud Centre / University College London, where he is also Programme Director for the MSc in Developmental Psychology and Clinical Practice.

Ioanna Vrouva is a Trainee Clinical Psychologist at University College London.

Minding the Child

Mentalization-based interventions with children, young people and their families

Edited by
Nick Midgley and Ioanna Vrouva

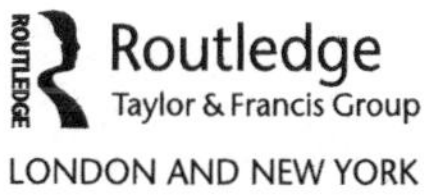

LONDON AND NEW YORK

First published 2012
by Routledge
27 Church Road, Hove, East Sussex BN3 2FA

Simultaneously published in the USA and Canada
by Routledge
711 Third Avenue, New York NY 10017

Routledge is an imprint of the Taylor & Francis Group, an Informa business

British Library Cataloguing in Publication Data
A catalogue record for this book is available from the British Library

Library of Congress Cataloging-in-Publication Data
Minding the child : mentalization-based interventions with children, young people, and their families / edited by Nick Midgley, Ioanna Vrouva.
p. cm.
Includes bibliographical references and index.
ISBN 978-0-415-60523-6 (hardback) – ISBN 978-0-415-60525-0 (soft cover) 1. Child psychotherapy. 2. Family psychotherapy. I. Midgley, Nick, 1968- II. Vrouva, Ioanna.
RJ504.M56 2012
618.92'8914–dc23

2011039547

ISBN: 978-0-415-60523-6 (hbk)
ISBN: 978-0-415-60525-0 (pbk)
ISBN: 978-0-203-12300-3 (ebk)

Typeset in Times by Garfield Morgan, Swansea, West Glamorgan
Paperback cover design by Andrew Ward

Contents

Contributors vii

Foreword xi
LINDA C. MAYES

Acknowledgements xiii

Introduction 1
NICK MIDGLEY AND IOANNA VROUVA

PART I
The concept of 'mentalization': theory and research 9

1 What is mentalization? The concept and its foundations in developmental research 11
PETER FONAGY AND ELIZABETH ALLISON

2 Mentalizing problems in children and adolescents 35
CARLA SHARP AND AMANDA VENTA

3 Measuring mentalization in children and young people 54
IOANNA VROUVA, MARY TARGET AND KARIN ENSINK

PART II
Clinic-based interventions 77

4 Mentalization-based treatment for parents (MBT-P) with borderline personality disorder and their infants 79
LIESBET NIJSSENS, PATRICK LUYTEN AND DAWN L. BALES

5 Minding the family mind: The development and initial evaluation of mentalization-based treatment for families 98
EMMA KEAVENY, NICK MIDGLEY, EIA ASEN, DICKON BEVINGTON, PASCO FEARON, PETER FONAGY, RUTH JENNINGS-HOBBS AND SALLY WOOD

6 Mentalization-based therapies with adopted children and their families 113
NICOLE MULLER, LIDEWIJ GERITS AND IRMA SIECKER

7 Self-harm in young people: Is MBT the answer? 131
TRUDIE ROSSOUW

PART III
Community-based interventions 145

8 Thinking and feeling in the context of chronic illness: A mentalization-based group intervention with adolescents 147
NORKA T. MALBERG

9 Supporting and enhancing mentalization in community outreach teams working with hard-to-reach youth: The AMBIT approach 163
DICKON BEVINGTON AND PETER FUGGLE

10 A developmental approach to mentalizing communities through the Peaceful Schools experiment 187
STUART W. TWEMLOW, PETER FONAGY AND FRANK C. SACCO

11 'Thoughts in mind': Promoting mentalizing communities for children 202
POUL LUNDGAARD BAK

Index 219

Contributors

Elizabeth Allison is a Psychoanalyst, an Honorary Senior Research Fellow in the Psychoanalysis Unit at University College London and a Senior Publications Editor at the Anna Freud Centre. She received her doctorate from Oxford University and her current research interests include the application of psychoanalytic ideas to the study of literature.

Eia Asen, MD, FRCPsych works as a Consultant Child and Adolescent Psychiatrist, as well as a Consultant Psychiatrist in Psychotherapy. He is the clinical director of the Marlborough Family Service in Central London and a Visiting Professor at University College London. He has authored and co-authored nine books, as well as many book chapters and scientific papers, mostly on working with families.

Dawn L. Bales is a clinical psychologist and psychotherapist, MBT trainer and supervisor. She works as the director of the expertise centre MBT in the Netherlands and does MBT research for the Viersprong Institute for Studies on Personality Disorders (VISPD).

Dickon Bevington is a Consultant in Child and Adolescent Psychiatry, working in Cambridgeshire and Peterborough NHS Foundation Trust. He also works in London at the Anna Freud Centre, where he co-leads (with Peter Fuggle) the AMBIT project and is part of the MBT-F team.

Karin Ensink, PhD is Associate Professor of Child and Adolescent Psychology at Laval University, Québec, Canada. Since completing her PhD on children's mentalization, she has been teaching modern psychodynamic approaches to the treatment and assessment of children and adolescents and conducts research on mentalization, attachment, trauma and personality in children and parents.

Pasco Fearon is Professor of Developmental Psychopathology at University College London and joint Director of the UCL Doctoral Programme in Clinical Psychology. His research focuses on early child development and particularly the role of attachment in risk for emotional and behavioural problems. His research is multidisciplinary, integrating traditional developmental and clinical psychology with methods from behavioural genetics and neuroscience. He is also the Director of the Anna Freud Centre's Developmental Neuroscience lab, and a visiting member of the faculty at the Child Study Center at Yale University.

Peter Fonagy, PhD, FBA is Freud Memorial Professor of Psychoanalysis and Head of the Research Department of Clinical, Educational and Health Psychology at University College London; Chief Executive of the Anna Freud Centre, London; and Consultant to the Child and Family Programme at the Menninger Department of Psychiatry and Behavioral Sciences at the Baylor College of Medicine.

Peter Fuggle is a Clinical Psychologist and Clinical Director of the Islington Child and Adolescent Mental Health Service in London. Since April 2008 he has also worked at the Anna Freud Centre, both as Course Director of the CBT for Children and Young People Masters course and as Training Advisor for the Centre.

Lidewij Gerits is a child and adolescent psychotherapist. She is specialized in MBT play therapy and MBT group therapy. She worked for several years in an outpatient MBT treatment programme for adolescents with emerging personality disorder and their families and worked with adoptive children. She runs courses in MBT and now works in a private practice in Leiden, the Netherlands.

Ruth Jennings-Hobbs is an Assistant Psychologist at the Anna Freud Centre, London, where she evaluates therapeutic services. She co-supervises the research projects of postgraduate psychology students at UCL and she has a Masters (Distinction) in Developmental Psychopathology from Durham University.

Emma Keaveny is a Clinical Psychologist in the Parent Consultation Service and Mentalization-Based Treatment for Families team at the Anna Freud Centre, London. She also works part-time as a Clinical Tutor and Lecturer at Royal Holloway, University of London on their Doctorate in Clinical Psychology Course.

Poul Lundgaard Bak is a Senior Researcher in Child Mental Health, currently working at the Institute of Public Health, Aarhus University. He obtained his MD in 1980 and has 25 years' experience in public health care and child health education.

Patrick Luyten, PhD is Professor at the Department of Psychology, University of Leuven; Senior Lecturer at the Research Department of Clinical, Educational, and Health Psychology at University College

London; and Adjunct Assistant Professor at the Yale Child Study Center, New Haven (USA).

Norka T. Malberg, MS, EdM, MsC, DPsych is a Child and Adolescent Psychotherapist trained at the Anna Freud Centre. She is currently in private practice in New Haven, Connecticut. Norka is one of the editors of the book, *The Anna Freudian Tradition: Lines of Development – Evolution of Theory and Practice over the Decades* (Karnac, 2011).

Nick Midgley is a child and adolescent psychotherapist and Director of Programme for the MSc in Developmental Psychology and Clinical Practice at the Anna Freud Centre/University College London. He is the joint editor of *Child Psychotherapy and Research: New Directions, Emerging Findings* (Routledge, 2009).

Nicole Muller is a child and adolescent psychotherapist and a family therapist. She has written several articles on MBT-F and MBT in the Netherlands and has translated the MBT-F protocol in Dutch (with C. ten Kate). She works at The Jutters, in the city of The Hague, in an outpatient and inpatient MBT treatment programme for children and adolescents with attachment and/or emerging personality disorders.

Liesbet Nijssens is a child psychologist and psychoanalytic psychotherapist. She works as a psychotherapist at the Mentalization-Based Treatment (MBT) unit at the Center of Psychotherapy De Viersprong, Halsteren (The Netherlands), and is a PhD student at the Department of Psychology, University of Leuven.

Trudie Rossouw is a consultant child and adolescent psychiatrist in the North East London Foundation Trust. She is a trained psychoanalyst and is associate medical director of the specialist services directorate.

Frank C. Sacco, PhD is President of Community Services Institute, Boston and Springfield, Massachusetts, a mental health center and pre-doctoral psychology internship training programme. He is an adjunct professor of psychology at Western New England College, Springfield, Massachusetts and Vice President of the International Association of Applied Psychoanalytic Studies.

Carla Sharp, PhD is an Associate Professor in the Department of Psychology at the University of Houston and Director of the Developmental Psychopathology Lab. Her research broadly focuses on the early identification of psychiatric disorder in youth, primarily through examining the role of social cognition.

Irma Siecker is a family therapist, specialised in MBT-F. She works in the Mental Health Centre for Children and Adolescents of Rivierduinen, Holland, with adoptive children and their families and in an outpatient

MBT-treatment programme for adolescents with emerging personality disorder and their families.

Mary Target, PhD, is Professor of Psychoanalysis at University College London, a Fellow of the British Psycho-Analytical Society and Professional Director of the Anna Freud Centre. She has researched attachment and psychotherapy outcome and is a Principal Investigator on four current projects.

Stuart W. Twemlow, MD is Professor of Psychiatry & Behavioral Sciences in the Menninger Department of Psychiatry, Baylor College of Medicine, Houston, TX, and is Senior Psychiatrist at the Menninger Clinic. His primary clinical and research focus is on innovative interventions to reduce violence and improve wellbeing in complex social systems including schools.

Amanda Venta, BA is a graduate student in the Clinical Psychology Programme of the University of Houston. Her research interests focus on social cognition, especially in the context of the parent–child relationship.

Ioanna Vrouva is a Trainee Clinical Psychologist at University College London. Funded by the Greek State Scholarship, she obtained a PhD from UCL. Prior to this, she completed an MSc (Distinct.) in Research Methods in Psychology at UCL, and a first class degree in Psychology at the National University of Athens.

Sally Wood is a Family Therapist at the Anna Freud Centre working in the MBT-F Team. Sally has a particular interest in integrating systemic and psychoanalytic work and working with looked after and adopted children and their families.

Foreword

Linda C. Mayes, MD

Yale Child Study Center, New Haven, CT and Anna Freud Centre, London

Trying to understand the why and how of human behaviour in our day-to-day lives draws us into wondering about the thoughts, feelings, and desires of ourselves and others. These are those states of mind we never really know with certainty, but which we sense are the 'Rosetta stone' for capturing the essence of what it means to be engaged in interactions with another person – whether in a caring, loving, hateful or even dismissive way. Some of the greatest tragedies of human interaction occur when an individual misinterprets or is cut off from this language of mind and hence cannot fully grasp the many meanings of gestures of love, friendship or hostility. As if in a foreign land with no comprehension of the native language, such a person often struggles to understand their own emotions and feels alone even when surrounded by others.

Learning to speak and understand this universal language of humanity is at the heart of this book. While writers and poets chronicle the tragedies of being 'mind blind', therapists whose currency is the language of thoughts, feelings, and desires take a creative approach to helping their patients become more curious and more fluent about the many ways to understand a single action.

Mentalization-based therapies have grown out of several intellectual and therapeutic traditions including the philosophy of mind, attachment theory and psychoanalysis. Each of the therapeutic approaches presented in this volume represents an effort both to understand how such a basic human capacity and need can be derailed, and also to develop innovative and effective ways to restore and strengthen an individual's capacity to reflect upon their own and others' thoughts, feelings, and desires. By doing so, these interventions aim to help children and families see new paths, to break out of habitual ways of being and acting. Most hopeful is the possibility that enhancing mentalization abilities in children facing challenges, such as chronic medical illness or severe family disruption, gives them a new set of life skills. Such skills are nurtured through more sustained and caring interactions with others in their expanded social world.

A special, fertile climate has fostered the innovative approaches presented in this book. The authors represented in this volume come from the world of academic developmental science as well as ongoing clinical work in schools, clinics, community centres and consulting rooms. They are brought together by collaborations with clinicians and scholars at the Anna Freud Centre, an institution with a longstanding commitment to bringing individuals together from different national and international settings with a shared focus on supporting children's emotional well-being through innovative training, scholarship and clinical approaches. The creativity exemplified by the intervention models in this book reflects what can happen when an institution facilitates conferences, trainings, and collaborations among creative individuals able to see new ways to take complex theories of mind and translate these into practical and effective treatments for children and their families. May this volume continue to foster innovation on behalf of children and their families in all those who read and adapt the work of its authors to their own settings.

Acknowledgements

The idea for this book was inspired by two conferences that took place in 2010 on the topic of mentalization-based interventions with children, young people and families – the first at the Anna Freud Centre in London, and the second at the Yale Child Study Centre in the USA. Although this volume is not a collection of papers from those conferences, many of the speakers at those events went on to contribute to this book; and the energy and excitement generated at those conferences inspired us to try and put something into print. We would like to thank all those who contributed to making those events such a success, not least those who helped organize the conferences, especially Wendy Smith (London) and Linda Isakower (Yale).

Thanks also go to Emily Gough, who helped us get our manuscript into shape; and to our editors at Routledge, Joanne Forshaw and Jane Harris, for supporting this project and answering all our queries so efficiently as the project progressed. Thanks also to the Guilford Press, for permission to reproduce the chapter by Stuart Twemlow *et al.*, originally published in the *Bulletin of the Menninger Clinic*; and to Prof. Simon Baron Cohen, for permission to reproduce an image from his 'Mind in the Eyes' test in Chapter 3. Special thanks for Kiriko Kubo for giving us permission to use her artwork as part of the cover design – and for so much more.

Introduction

Mentalization-based interventions for children, young people and families

Nick Midgley and Ioanna Vrouva

The concept of 'mentalization' is both a relatively new one and an extremely old one. It has been described as 'a form of imaginative mental activity, namely, perceiving and interpreting human behaviour in terms of intentional mental states (e.g. needs, desires, feelings, beliefs, goals, purposes, and reasons)' (Fonagy *et al.*, 2002). Over the last 20 years or so, a small group of gifted clinicians and scholars have gradually elucidated the various aspects of this concept, making a strong case for seeing the capacity to mentalize as a fundamental component of what it means to be human. As well as playing a central role in the emergence of affect regulation and the development of a coherent sense of self (Fonagy *et al.*, 2002), these authors also propose that the capacity to reflect on the mental states of self and others is central to the process of therapeutic change across a range of treatments, and is therefore the legitimate focus of more targeted clinical interventions (Allen *et al.*, 2008).

Largely rooted in the field of developmental research and with conceptual origins in both psychoanalysis and attachment theory, mentalization – and the empirical research which has supported it – has provided a rich set of ideas about the development of the self and the ability to relate with others, the way in which attachment disruption and trauma impact on our capacity to think about our own minds and the minds of others, and the ways in which this capacity can be fostered in a therapeutic relationship with an explicit focus on mentalization. The study of mentalization has from the very beginning been an 'applied' science, developing not just from work in the laboratory, but also from clinical practice.

Mentalization-based treatment (MBT) is now an evidence-based approach for working with people diagnosed with borderline personality disorder (BPD, Bateman & Fonagy, 2004, 2006) and this model of therapy is becoming increasingly widespread. However, despite the fact that the concept of mentalization has its roots in developmental theory and science – and that some of the key clinical concepts emerged out of therapeutic work with children (e.g. Fonagy & Moran, 1991; Hurry, 1998) – to date there has been less attention paid to the implications of the concept of mentalization for work with children, young people and their families. So too, adaptations of mentalization-based treatment have not yet established themselves as evidence-based approaches to working with young people and their families in the same way that they have begun to do in work with adults.

The main aim of this book is to provide an introduction to the concept of mentalization and to make a case for its relevance for work with children, young people and their families. But clinical models from an adult setting do not automatically translate across to work with young people, and in this book our aim is not so much to present a single model of MBT for young people, but rather to introduce a range of applications of mentalizing ideas to existing ways of working with young people. Indeed, we hope the chapters in this book will show that mentalization-enhancing interventions can be a useful refinement of most psychosocial treatments. This is because attending to mental states in oneself and others is a fundamental common factor inherent in any psychotherapeutic work (Allen *et al.*, 2008).

Just as clinicians from a broad spectrum of schools of therapy (including interpersonal psychotherapy, psychodynamic, cognitive, systemic and client-centred therapy) have embraced ideas about mentalizing as a way to enhance their work with adults, likewise child and adolescent mental health professionals from a range of backgrounds are now beginning to grasp the broader significance of mentalization and to creatively integrate it with their own modalities. Pioneers such as Verheugt-Pleiter *et al.* (2008) demonstrated the role of mentalizing in child therapy, and now colleagues from around the world are taking these ideas forward in a range of different settings. What brings all these different approaches together, we believe, is the commitment to understanding subjectivity in a relational context, and recognizing the importance of 'keeping the child's mind in mind'.

Primarily, the book is intended as a practical clinical text for those working with children, young people and their families in the mental health field; we hope that both novice and experienced clinicians will be able to enhance their knowledge and practice through the pages that follow. In most cases, the work described in this book is carried out by professionals who already have core therapeutic training and skills for working with young people and their families, and the mentalizing focus is seen as an additional element to existing skills. Some of the chapters, however, also show how ideas about mentalizing can be adapted outside the clinical setting, and may be of relevance to those with no prior mental health training, but with a real commitment to supporting children's development through paying attention to their minds.

Drawing from a wide range of sources, we hope that those who are not clinicians will also find this volume of interest, including policymakers, teachers, social workers, foster carers and parents. Research psychologists and developmentalists from other disciplines may also be interested in how the ideas described in the book link theory with practice.

The overall organization of the book is relatively straightforward: Part I is primarily theoretical and aims to provide an overview of the concept of mentalization; in Part II we introduce a range of settings in which mentalization-based interventions have been developed to work with children and young people in child mental health services; and in Part III we introduce a number of adaptations of mentalizing ideas to work with young people and their families in community settings. Each chapter focuses on work with different ages (parents and babies, children and families, adolescents), using different formats (individual, family or group) and delivered in different settings (mental health clinics, schools, hospitals, etc.).

Part I of the book has three chapters, and begins with an overview of the concept of mentalization and its foundations in developmental research, written by Peter Fonagy and Elizabeth Allison. The authors provide a summary of the development of mentalization and its main characteristics and they outline a developmental model of mentalization drawing on attachment theory. This is followed by a chapter by Carla Sharp and Amanda Venta, which provides an overview of the research literature on the mentalizing problems associated with each major class of psychiatric disorder in childhood (developmental, externalizing and internalizing disorders). In reviewing the literature, the authors (a) establish mentalizing as an important endophenotype to be targeted in treatment and (b) illuminate how different aspects of mentalizing are reflected in the heterogeneity of different childhood disorders.

The importance of targeting and measuring specific mechanisms of change (like mentalizing) in treatment outcome studies is emphasized by Sharp and Venta, which leads neatly into the third and final chapter in the opening section of the book. If the capacity to mentalize is posited as an important target for therapeutic interventions, it is essential that researchers are able to find ways of measuring children's capacities to mentalize. Yet there are many obstacles to developing reliable and valid measures of this multifaceted and mercurial capacity. Part I therefore ends with a chapter by Ioanna Vrouva, Mary Target and Karin Ensink, outlining some emerging methods of assessing mentalization in children and adolescents. The authors raise some important points about the difficulties of 'measuring' mentalization, and discuss some of the ways in which this has been attempted so far.

Taken together, we hope that the chapters in Part I of the book will give the reader who has little familiarity with the concept of mentalization an understanding of the concept, where the concept comes from and why it matters. The reader will also get an idea of the latest research into the role of mentalizing in a range of childhood disorders and a picture of some of the creative ways in which researchers are now trying to measure this important capacity, which can change so rapidly from moment to moment and from one developmental stage to the next. For those already familiar with this literature, we hope these chapters will still serve as a useful gathering together of what we do (and don't) know; but those readers may prefer to move directly to Part II of the book.

Part II introduces four different models of clinic-based therapy for children, all drawing in different but related ways on ideas about mentalizing. The chapters range from interventions with parents and babies to individual therapy, focusing on different clinical populations and describing a variety of treatment formats. In Chapter 4, Liesbet Nijssens, Patrick Luyten and Dawn Bales discuss mentalization-based treatment for parents (MBT-P), a therapeutic approach which builds on MBT principles, but is specifically tailored to the needs of parents with borderline personality disorder (BPD) who have children between the ages of 0 and 4. This chapter describes the theoretical underpinnings, the key intervention principles and structure of MBT-P, as well as current ongoing research concerning the efficacy of this model of working.

In the following chapter, Emma Keaveny and her colleagues describe the development and initial evaluation of a mentalization-based treatment for families (MBT-F) service at the Anna Freud Centre, London. This chapter discusses clinical work that aims at increasing the mentalizing capacity of whole families, supporting them to clarify the specific thoughts, feelings, wishes and beliefs which underpin each other's habitual attitudes and behaviours. As with all the clinical contributions in this book, the chapter provides a number of clinical examples of some of the key aspects of MBT-F, and also describes a new approach to manualizing treatment that has been piloted in the Anna Freud Centre's MBT-F service – the 'wiki-manual'.

In Chapter 6, Nicole Muller and her colleagues from The Jutters Clinic in the Netherlands give an account of their team's work with families with adopted children using MBT-F, often in combination with MBT play therapy for the child. They describe their attempts at overcoming the difficult problems these families often encounter, focusing especially on moments of high emotion within adoptive families which might inhibit the capacity to mentalize successfully about the behaviour and feelings of one's self and of others. They describe a characteristic existential vulnerability that adopted children often have to deal with. Questions like 'Do I have the right to live?', 'Why was I given away?', 'Do my parents love me?' are topics that often arise in therapy. The authors show how a mentalizing approach, where family members learn to be aware of their inner feelings and thoughts, can help with the severe strains that these families often experience.

Part II ends with a chapter by Trudie Rossouw in which she describes a research study that tried to examine whether difficulties with mentalizing may be a significant factor for adolescents who self-harm. Based on this research study, Rossouw and her colleagues went on to develop and evaluate an adaptation of MBT for working with this very vulnerable population. The research that Trudie Rossouw describes in Chapter 7 began as a cross-sectional analysis comparing a group of adolescents who self-harm against two control groups on a variety of clinical, cognitive and psychosocial dimensions. The group presenting with self-harm was concurrently enrolled into a randomized controlled trial (RCT) comparing mentalization-based treatment for adolescents (MBT-A) and treatment as usual (TAU). The RCT is still underway, but this chapter provides some intriguing results of the initial cross-sectional analysis along with an outline of the MBT treatment model as it has been adapted to work with this group of young people.

The chapters in Part II of the book show a range of creative ways in which clinicians have adapted and adopted ideas from MBT for use with young people and their families who are engaging with mental health services. But one of the characteristics of mentalization-based interventions is their flexibility and adaptability in different settings. So Part III focuses on community-based interventions in a range of settings, shifting towards prevention and early intervention and mobilizing communities to use their own mentalizing resources to prevent difficulties from developing.

In Chapter 8, Norka Malberg describes the development of a mentalization-based group intervention within a paediatric haemodialysis unit at Great Ormond Street Hospital, London. The chapter gives detailed examples of interactions during the process of setting up and implementing the group, and the author emphasizes the importance of working with the diverse systems within the hospital unit and of considering variables such as cultural values and beliefs. Results of the intervention are briefly outlined and Malberg demonstrates the particular contribution that she feels a mentalizing stance can offer to young people with significant health problems as well as the health professionals who work with them.

Whilst a hospital is a relatively self-contained setting, many services are attempting to work with very 'hard-to-reach' populations, where simply engaging the young people may be a major challenge to any kind of work. In Chapter 9, Dickon Bevington and Peter Fuggle describe an approach they have developed at the Anna Freud Centre called Adolescent Mentalization-Based Integrative Therapy (AMBIT). They make the case that mentalization provides a helpful integrative framework for the multidisciplinary context in which most work with multiply troubled, complex, high risk, hard-to-reach youth is located. The authors argue that in a hard-to-reach youth population, the conventional professional system's response has sometimes been to multiply the number of professionals involved (often in proportion to the perceived risks). In contrast, they argue that this can be counterproductive, as the young person is confronted with multiple conversations, frequently appearing contradictory, which easily become overpowering and aversive. Instead, they suggest that a multimodally trained key worker, focusing on the development of a therapeutically effective attachment relationship, and powerfully supported by a well-connected team, may act as a more potent agent for change. The authors show how such workers can be supported not only to work with mentalizing as a therapeutic tool with individuals and their families, but also to use it as the framework for innovative and robust processes of supervision. These are interventions aimed at identifying and repairing the inevitable 'dis-integrations' that occur in the multi-agency context of any such work.

The last two chapters in this section focus on schools, which play such an important role in the lives of children and young people. In Chapter 10, Stuart Twemlow and his colleagues describe a developmental approach to mentalizing communities, through the Peaceful Schools experiment. This chapter contrasts a social systems approach to school bullying and violence with a mentalization approach to the same problem, and then attempts a synthesis of the two. The authors propose that the serious contemporary problem of bullying and interpersonal violence in schools could be better approached using a focus on the relationships between the members of the social system as a whole, rather than the more traditional strategy seen in prevention studies, i.e. that of identifying disturbed and at risk children and separating them from the social system for special attention. The chapter then outlines a set of steps that might be necessary to create 'mentalizing schools' that have a sophisticated developmental focus on the individual needs of the members as reflected in the conduct of the system as a whole. Finally, the authors provide a brief summary of the findings of a test of these ideas in a randomized controlled trial in the USA involving several schools and over 3000 children.

The final chapter in this section describes a project called Thoughts in Mind (TiM), a school-based education programme developed in Denmark. TiM is a community-based psychoeducational programme which aims to educate parents and teachers in how to how to use 'mentalizing ideas' in their day-to-day interactions with children, as an integral part of daily life and regular activities. The author describes TiM as 'practical knowledge vitamins about thoughts, feelings and the brain' for adults who spend time with children and adolescents. This last chapter brings us back full circle to the theory of mentalizing presented in Chapter 1 by Fonagy and Allison – but now presented in a very different way. A crucial core of the TiM project is to translate scientific theory and knowledge about mentalization into practical knowledge at 'children's height' (in narrative, images and metaphors) – within a realistic time and resource framework.

Taken together, we hope that these chapters give a sense of the range and creativity of the work currently being developed for children and families under the umbrella of 'mentalization-based interventions'. Readers will notice that in almost all the chapters describing the development of new interventions there has been a commitment to empirical evaluation. This is indeed another crucial aspect of the mentalizing approach, as empirical evaluation presupposes a 'not knowing' stance and expresses a genuine interest in the other's experience. Committed to practicing what they preach, the authors also invite readers in a lively and accessible way to their research labs, therapy sessions and community projects throughout the book, by including various examples, vignettes and case histories. In order to prevent identification, the names and identifiable details of the people presented have been changed, or in some descriptions a number of cases have been combined, in order to protect the confidentiality of the young people and families involved.

From inception to completion this book was supported by the Anna Freud Centre in London, a Centre of Practice and Learning committed to understanding and supporting children's emotional well-being through innovative research, training and clinical services. Most of the book contributors have been participants in conferences and clinical seminars on mentalizing held at the Anna Freud Centre and it is their enthusiasm and creativity that has led to the development of new services in the UK and abroad. However, these services are by no means the only model of how things could be done. We anticipate (and hope) that readers will find their own imaginative ways to further elaborate the practices described in this book, and adapt what is presented here to their own particular work context, and to the needs and aspirations of the young people and families with whom they work.

References

Allen, J., Fonagy, P., & Bateman, A. (2008). *Mentalizing in clinical practice*. Washington, DC: American Psychiatric Press.

Bateman, A., & Fonagy, P. (2004). Mentalization-based treatment for borderline personality disorder. *Journal of Personality Disorders*, 18(1), 36–51.

Bateman, A., & Fonagy, P. (2006). *Mentalization-based treatment for borderline personality disorder: A practical guide*. Oxford: Oxford University Press.

Fonagy, P., & Moran, G.S. (1991). Understanding psychic change in child psychoanalysis. *International Journal of Psycho-Analysis*, 72, 15–22.

Fonagy, P., Gergely, G., Jurist, E., & Target, M. (2002). *Affect regulation, mentalization and the development of the self*. New York: Other Press.

Hurry, A. (1998). *Psychoanalysis and developmental therapy*. London: Karnac.

Verheugt-Pleiter, A., Zevalkink, J., & Schmeets, M. (Eds.) (2008). *Mentalizing in child therapy: Guidelines for clinical practitioners*. London: Karnac.

Part I

The concept of 'mentalization': theory and research

Chapter 1

What is mentalization?

The concept and its foundations in developmental research

Peter Fonagy and Elizabeth Allison

Introduction: What is mentalization?

When we mentalize we are engaged in a form of (mostly preconscious) imaginative mental activity that enables us to perceive and interpret human behaviour in terms of intentional mental states, e.g. needs, desires, feelings, beliefs, goals, purposes and reasons (Allen *et al.*, 2008). Mentalizing must be imaginative because we have to imagine what other people might be thinking or feeling. We can never know for sure what is in someone else's mind (Fonagy *et al.*, 1997b). Moreover, we suggest (perhaps counter-intuitively) that a similar kind of imaginative leap is required to understand our own mental experience, particularly in relation to emotionally charged issues. We shall see that the ability to mentalize is vital for self-organization and affect regulation.

The ability to infer and represent other people's mental states may be uniquely human. It seems to have evolved to enable humans to predict and interpret others' actions quickly and efficiently in a large variety of competitive and cooperative situations. However, the extent to which each of us is able to master this vital capacity is crucially influenced by our early experiences as well as our genetic inheritance. In this chapter, we discuss the evolutionary function of attachment relationships, arguing that their major evolutionary advantage is the opportunity that they give infants to develop social intelligence, as well as to acquire the capacity for affect regulation and attentional control. We review evidence from the developmental literature on the social influences on attachment and mentalization. We then describe how our understanding of ourselves and others as mental agents grows out of interpersonal experience, particularly the child–caregiver relationship (Fonagy *et al.*, 2002), and how the development of the ability to mentalize may be compromised in children who have not benefited from the opportunity to be understood and thought about in this way by a sensitive caregiver. Finally, we offer some reflections on the challenges of mentalizing in family interactions.

Origins of the concept of mentalization

We first developed our concept of mentalization in the context of a large empirical study, in which security of infant attachment with each parent turned out to be strongly predicted, not only by that parent's security of attachment during the pregnancy (Fonagy *et al.*, 1991a), but even more by the parent's ability to think about and understand their childhood relationship to their own parents in terms of states of mind (Fonagy *et al.*, 1991b). We proposed that there was a vital synergy between attachment processes and the development of the child's ability to understand interpersonal behaviour in terms of mental states (Fonagy *et al.*, 1997a, 2002).

Alongside this empirical research, inspiration for the development of the concept of mentalization also came from psychoanalytic work with borderline patients. In an early paper effectively co-authored with George Moran, we identified the repudiation of a concern with mental states as a key aspect of borderline psychopathology (Fonagy, 1991). The first time we used the term mentalization was in 1989 (Fonagy, 1989), influenced by the Ecole Psychosomatique de Paris, but we used the term as operationalized by developmental researchers investigating theory of mind (ToM; Leslie, 1987). The failure of mentalizing had of course been apparent to most psychoanalysts working with these patients, particularly Bion, Rosenfeld, Green, Kernberg and the North American object relations theorists. In an early paper reviewing ideas concerning mentalization in relation to classical psychoanalytic concepts, this intellectual indebtedness was carefully documented (Fonagy & Higgitt, 1989). The basic suggestion was that the capacity for representing self and others as thinking, believing, wishing or desiring does not simply arrive at age four, as an inevitable consequence of maturation. Rather, it is a developmental achievement that is profoundly rooted in the quality of early relationships. Its liability to disappear under stress in borderline conditions was seen as an appropriate focus for psychoanalytically oriented psychological intervention.

A second line of analytic inspiration came from work with children undertaken as part of a project to construct a manual for child analysis and subsequent work in developmental science by Mary Target and Peter Fonagy (Fonagy *et al.*, 2002; Fonagy & Target, 1996, 2000, 2007; Target & Fonagy, 1996). This work helped us to think more deeply about the normal development of thinking or mentalizing capacity, and the more primitive modes of thought that precede its emergence. In trying to map the emergence of mentalization on the basis of material from records of child analysis and clinical and research work with children in other contexts, we came up with a heuristic map of the emergence of mentalization that turned out to be extremely valuable in understanding some qualitative aspects of the thinking of patients in borderline states. In particular, we noticed that the types of thinking that many have identified as a hallmark of borderline personality disorder were not dissimilar to the ways young children normally tend to treat their internal experience.

Our theory of the developmental emergence of the capacity to mentalize challenges the Cartesian assumption that the mind is transparent to itself and that our ability to reflect on our own minds is innate. We contend that optimal development of the capacity to mentalize depends on interaction with more mature and sensitive minds, and thus a consideration of the role played by attachment in this development is indispensable. We have come to conceive of mentalization as a multidimensional construct, whose core processing dimensions are underpinned by distinct neural systems. Thus, mentalization involves both a self-reflective and an interpersonal component; it is based both on observing others and reflecting on their mental states, it is both implicit and explicit and concerns both feelings and cognitions (Fonagy & Luyten, 2009; Lieberman, 2007; Luyten *et al.*, submitted; Saxe, 2006). When they are working together in optimal combination, the neural systems underpinning these components enable the child to represent causal mental states, distinguish inner from outer reality, infer others' mental states from subtle behavioural and contextual cues, moderate behaviour and emotional experience and construct representations of his or her own mental states from perceptible cues (arousal, behaviour or context).

Attachment and mentalization

Early caregiving relationships are probably key to normal development in all mammals, including humans (Hofer, 1995). John Bowlby, the founder of attachment theory, postulated a universal human need to form close bonds. Bowlby originally proposed that the basic evolutionary function of the attachment instinct was to ensure that infants would be protected from predators (Bowlby, 1969). The baby's attachment behaviours (e.g. proximity seeking, smiling, clinging) are reciprocated by adult attachment behaviours (touching, holding, soothing) and these responses reinforce the baby's attachment behaviour toward that particular adult.

However, the evolutionary role of the attachment relationship goes far beyond giving physical protection to the human infant. The infant's attachment behaviours are activated when something about his environment makes him feel insecure. The goal of the attachment system is an experience of security. Thus, the attachment system is first and foremost a regulator of emotional experience (Sroufe, 1996).

None of us are born with the capacity to regulate our own emotional reactions. As the caregiver understands and responds to the newborn infant's signals of moment-to-moment changes in his state, a dyadic regulatory system gradually evolves. The infant learns that he will not be overwhelmed by his emotional arousal while he is in the caregiver's presence, because the caregiver is there to help him re-establish equilibrium. Thus, when he starts to feel overwhelmed, he will seek or signal to the caregiver in the hope of soothing and the recovery of homeostasis. By the end of the first year, the infant's behaviour seems to be based on specific expectations. His past experiences with the caregiver are aggregated into representational systems which Bowlby (1973) termed 'internal working models' (IWMs).

Bowlby proposed that the IWMs of the self and others established in infancy provide prototypes for all later relationships. Because IWMs function outside of awareness, they are change-resistant (Crittenden, 1990). The stability of attachment has been demonstrated by longitudinal studies of infants assessed with the Strange Situation (Ainsworth *et al.*, 1978) and followed up in adolescence or young adulthood with the Adult Attachment Interview (AAI, George *et al.*, 1985). Longitudinal studies have shown a 68 to 75 per cent correspondence between attachment classifications in infancy and classifications in adulthood (e.g. Main, 1997). This is an unparalleled level of consistency between behaviour observed in infancy and outcomes in adulthood, although it is important to remember that such behaviour may be maintained by consistent environments as well as by patterns laid down in the first year of life.

Attachment relationships also play a key role in the transgenerational transmission of security. Secure adults are three or four times more likely to have children who are securely attached to them (van IJzendoorn, 1995). One might wonder if such powerful intergenerational effects are genetically mediated, but evidence from behaviour genetic studies offers no support for genetic transmission (e.g. Fearon *et al.*, 2006). Parental attachment patterns predict unique variance in addition to temperament measures or contextual factors, such as life events, social support and psychopathology (Steele *et al.*, unpublished manuscript). However, the precise mechanisms which ensure that securely attached mothers and fathers develop secure attachment relationships with their child have been difficult to identify (van IJzendoorn, 1995).

Insecure infant attachment, and particularly disorganized attachment, is a risk factor for suboptimal emotional and social development (Lyons-Ruth & Jacobvitz, 2008). But accumulating evidence shows that the developmental pathway from disorganized infant attachment to later psychological disorder is complex and sometimes circuitous. Rather than a developmentally reductionist model, moving directly from infancy to adulthood, we must envision a complex series of steps, each involving factors of risk and resilience interacting with past and future developmental phases. However, infant attachment may be a vulnerability factor that can illuminate the entire developmental process.

In our view, the major evolutionary advantage of attachment in humans is the opportunity it gives the infant to develop social intelligence. Alan

Sroufe (1996) and Myron Hofer (2004) played a seminal role in extending the scope of attachment theory from an account of the developmental emergence of a set of social expectations, to a far broader conception of attachment as an organizer of physiological and brain regulation. Attachment ensures that the brain processes which serve social cognition are appropriately organized and prepared to enable us to live and work with other people.

There is increasing evidence suggesting that the formation of attachment relationships is supported by at least two neurobiological systems: (1) linking attachment experiences to reward and pleasure, motivating the caregiver (and in all likelihood the infant as well) to seek experiences of closeness; and (2) a neurobiological system linking enhanced social understanding to the attachment context, with closer bonds triggering biological systems that are likely to enhance sensitivity to social cues. Given the availability of a neurobiological pathway, what can the developmental psychology literature tell us about the link between attachment and mentalization?

Understanding the relationship of attachment and mentalization

If attachment underpins the emergence of mentalization we would expect secure children to outperform insecure ones in this domain (measured as passing ToM tasks earlier). Many studies support this hypothesis (see Fonagy & Luyten, 2009 for a review). Generally it seems that secure attachment and mentalization may be subject to similar social influences. We briefly consider some of these influences below.

Mentalizing and parenting

Two decades of research have confirmed that parenting is the key determinant of attachment security. Can aspects of parenting account for the overlap between mentalization and attachment security? In particular, does parental mentalization of the child have an influence? The mother's capacity to think about her child's mind is variously called maternal mind-mindedness, insightfulness and reflective function (RF). These overlapping attributes appear to be associated with both secure attachment and mentalization in the child (see Sharp *et al.*, 2006).

Elizabeth Meins (Meins *et al.*, 2001), David Oppenheim (Oppenheim & Koren-Karie, 2002) and Arietta Slade (Slade *et al.*, 2005) have all been able to link parental mentalization of the infant with the development of affect regulation and secure attachment in the child, mostly by analysing interactional narratives between parents and children. Although Meins assessed parents' quality of narrative about their children in real time (i.e. while the parents were playing with their children) and Oppenheim's group did this in a more 'off-line' manner (parent narrating videotaped interaction), both concluded that maternal mentalizing was a more significant predictor of security of attachment than, say, global sensitivity. Slade and colleagues (Slade *et al.*, 2005) also observed a strong relationship between attachment in the infant and the quality of the parent's mentalizing about the child. Low mentalizing mothers were more likely to show atypical maternal behaviour on the Atypical Maternal Behavior Instrument for Assessment and Classification (AMBIANCE; Bronfman *et al.*, 1999), which relates not only to infant attachment disorganization but also to unresolved (disorganized) attachment status in the mother's Adult Attachment Interview (Grienenberger *et al.*, 2005).

Taken together, these results suggest that mentalizing parents might well facilitate the development of mentalization in their children. Mindful parenting probably enhances both attachment security and mentalization. However, we should bear in mind that while these correlations could be understood as parent-to-child effects, they can be just as readily explained as child-to-parent effects. For example, less power-assertive parenting may be associated with mentalization (Pears & Moses, 2003) not because this may facilitate independent thinking, but because less mentalizing children may be more likely to elicit controlling parenting behaviour. It may also be that the same aspects of family functioning that facilitate secure attachment also facilitate the emergence of mentalizing.

The process of acquiring mentalization is so ordinary and normal that it may be more appropriate to consider secure attachment as providing an environment that is free of obstacles to its development rather than providing active and direct facilitation. The key to understanding the interaction of attachment with the development of mentalization may then be to look at instances where normally available catalysts to the development of mentalization are absent.

Family discourse

Exposure to normal family conversations appears to be a precondition of mentalization (Siegal & Patterson, 2008). Nicaraguan deaf adults who grew up without hearing references to beliefs appear to be incapable of passing false belief tests – tests which assess a child's grasp of the concept that people can have mental states which do not correspond with reality in a straightforward way and that these 'false beliefs' can affect their behaviour (Pyers, 2003, cited in Siegal & Patterson, 2008). Under normal circumstances, conversations in which adults and children talk about the intentions implied by each other's reasonable comments and link these to each other's appropriately interpreted actions may be the 'royal road' to understanding minds. The groundbreaking work of Mary Main (Hill *et al.*,

2003) helps to generate explanatory schemas by means of which other people's behaviour can be understood and predicted.

Playfulness

Playfulness is another feature of a secure attachment context. Play may also be important in acquiring mentalizing. The impact of lack of playfulness is most obvious in extreme cases. Blind children's active pretend play is quite limited (Fraiberg, 1977) and they also understand pretend play poorly (Lewis *et al.*, 2000). They are delayed on false belief tests and only pass when they reach a verbal mental age of 11 as opposed to the more normal age five (McAlpine & Moore, 1985). Blind infants also miss out on access to non-verbal information about inner states. They are deprived of cues to internal states such as facial expression, and can experience problems of identity which are perhaps associated with mentalization problems (Hobson & Bishop, 2003).

Maltreatment

Maltreatment disorganizes the attachment system (see Cicchetti & Valentino, 2006 for a comprehensive review). Does it disrupt mentalization? The evidence for significant developmental delay in these children's understanding of emotions is consistent, if slightly reduced when IQ and SES are controlled for (e.g. Frodi & Smetana, 1984; Smith & Walden, 1999). In addition to problems of emotional understanding, social cognition deficits and delayed ToM understanding have been reported in maltreated children (e.g. Cicchetti *et al.*, 2003; Pears & Fisher, 2005).

The mentalization deficit associated with childhood maltreatment may be a form of decoupling, inhibition or even a phobic reaction to mentalizing. Maltreatment can contribute to an acquired, partial 'mind-blindness' by compromising open reflective communication between parent and child. It might undermine the benefit derived from learning about the links between internal states and actions in attachment relationships (e.g. the child may be told that they 'deserve', 'want' or even 'enjoy' the abuse). This will more obviously be destructive if the maltreatment is perpetrated by a family member. Even where this is not the case, the parents' lack of awareness that maltreatment is taking place outside the home may invalidate the child's communications with the parent about how the child is feeling. The child finds that reflective discourse does not correspond to his feelings, a consistent misunderstanding that could reduce the child's ability to understand/mentalize verbal explanations of other people's actions. In these circumstances, such children are likely to struggle to detect mental states behind actions accurately, and will tend to see actions as inevitable rather than intended. This may be further complicated by the internalization of the caregiver-figure: when children are regularly unable to 'find' themselves as intentional beings in the reflective stance of their actual caregiver, they have no choice but to internalize a representation of their caregiver into their self-representation. This inevitably disorganizes the self-structure, creating splits. It also gives rise to the well-recognized phenomena associated with disorganization of attachment, such as the manipulativeness in middle childhood which is characteristic of individuals whose attachment was disorganized in infancy (George & Solomon, 1999).

Manipulativeness (and oppositional behaviour) as a consequence of attachment disorganization occurs because the child prefers to externalize the alien part of the self by nudging the caregiver (gently and sometimes not so gently) to experience the angry or anxious states of mind that they have internalized, but experience as alien (Fonagy *et al.*, 2002). This creates a situation where the child's own unwanted mental states can be felt to belong to somebody else, enabling the individual with disorganized attachment history to experience a measure of self-coherence.

Maltreatment creates a further profound complication within this mechanism, when the child uses split-off parts of the self to gain illusory control over the abuser, a process that has been richly described in the psychoanalytic literature as identification with the aggressor (Freud, 1936). When the child internalizes the mental state of the victimizer into the alien part of the self, they experience a part of their own mind as torturing, bent on the destruction of the ego. This leads to an unbearably painful emotional state where the self is experienced as evil and hateful. In these circumstances, it may feel as though the only solution is to turn the attack from within the mind against the body by self-harming. Alternatively, the individual with a history of maltreatment may resort to constantly externalizing the alien, torturing parts of the self-structure into a person close by. Through projective identification (as best described by Rosenfeld, 1971) the persecutory parts of the self are located in someone else. In this way the need for the alien experiences to be owned by another mind may lead to their involvement in a sequence of further abusive relationships. The need for projective identification is a matter of life and death for those with a traumatizing part of the self-structure, but this constellation creates a dependence on the object that has many of the features of addiction.

It would be absurd to suggest (either from a scientific or a common-sense perspective) that positive attachment experience is the only relationship influence on the development of mentalization. Negative experiences (e.g. emotionally charged conflict) may as readily facilitate the rapid development of mentalizing as positive emotions that are linked with secure attachment (Newton *et al.*, 2000). The reality is that numerous aspects of relational influence are likely to be involved in the emergence of mentalizing, some of which probably correlate with secure attachment. But studies of social influence on mentalizing have hitherto mistakenly tended to assume that this social cognitive capacity is unimodal.

As we suggested above, mentalization is probably better considered as a complex multi-component capacity with a variety of determinants, some of which are genetic while others are more influenced by environmental interference and facilitation. Each of the correlates of secure attachment we considered above may interface with one or more of a series of a range of neuropsychologically defined components of mentalizing (see Fonagy & Luyten, 2009 for a review).

The development of an agentive self: the social acquisition of social cognition

If children's caregiving environments are the key to their development as social beings, how do these environmental influences have their effect? Our model relies on the child's innate capacity to detect aspects of his world that react contingently to his own actions. In his first months of life, the baby begins to understand that he is a physical agent whose actions can bring about changes in bodies with which he has immediate physical contact (Leslie, 1994). At the same time, he begins to understand that he is a social agent, as he learns that his behaviour affects his caregiver's behaviour and emotions (Neisser, 1988). Both these early forms of self-awareness probably evolve through the workings of an innate contingency detection mechanism that enables the infant to analyse the probability of causal links between his actions and stimulus events (Watson, 1994). The child's initial preoccupation with perfectly response-contingent stimulation (provided by the proprioceptive sensory feedback generated by his own actions) allows him to differentiate himself from his environment and to construct a primary representation of his bodily self.

At about three to four months, an infant's preference appears to change. At this stage, the infant begins to be drawn to high-but-imperfect contingencies rather than perfect contingency (Bahrick & Watson, 1985) – the level of contingency that characterizes an attuned caregiver's empathic mirroring responses to a baby's emotional displays. Repeated experience of these responses enables the baby to begin to differentiate his internal self-states: a process that has been termed 'social biofeedback' (Gergely & Watson, 1996). A congenial and secure attachment relationship vitally contributes to the emergence of early mentalizing capacities by allowing the infant to 'discover' or 'find' his or her psychological self in the social world (Gergely, 2001).

At first, infants are not introspectively aware of different emotion states. Instead, their representations of these emotions are primarily based on stimuli received from the external world. Babies learn to differentiate the internal patterns of physiological and visceral stimulation that accompany different emotions by observing their caregivers' facial or vocal mirroring responses to these (e.g. Legerstee & Varghese, 2001; Mitchell, 1993). The baby comes to associate his control over the parents' mirroring displays with the resulting improvement in his emotional state, and this lays the foundations for his eventual development of the capacity for emotional self-regulation. The establishment of a second-order representation of affect states creates the basis for affect regulation and impulse control: affects can be manipulated and discharged internally as well as through action, they can also be experienced as something recognizable and hence shared.

Two conditions need to be met if the capacity to understand and regulate emotions is to develop: (a) reasonable congruency of mirroring whereby the caregiver accurately matches the infant's mental state; and (b) 'markedness' of the mirroring, whereby the caregiver is able to express an affect while indicating that she is not expressing her own feelings (Gergely & Watson, 1999). If the caregiver's mirroring is incongruent, the resulting representation of the infant's internal state will not correspond to a constitutional self state, which might predispose the infant to develop a narcissistic personality structure (perhaps analogous to Winnicott's notion of a 'false self' – Winnicott, 1965). If the mirroring is unmarked, the caregiver's expression may seem to externalize the infant's experience and may overwhelm the infant, making his experience seem contagious and escalating rather than regulating his state. A predisposition to experiencing emotion through other people (as in a borderline personality structure) might then be established (Fonagy *et al.*, 2002).

Affect regulation, attentional control and mentalization

The child is thought to internalize his experience of well-regulated affect in the infant–parent couple to form the basis of a secure attachment bond and internal working model (Sroufe, 1996). In this account, affect regulation is a prelude to mentalization; yet, once mentalization occurs, the nature of affect regulation is transformed. Not only does mentalization allow adjustment of affect states but, more fundamentally, it is used to regulate the self. The emergence of mentalizing function follows a well-researched developmental line that identifies 'fixation points':

(a) *During the second half of the first year of life*, the child begins to be able to grasp the causal relations between actions, their agents and the environment. At around nine months, infants begin to look at actions in terms of the actor's underlying intentions (Baldwin *et al.*, 2001) and they begin to understand themselves as teleological agents who can choose the most efficient way to bring about a goal from a range of alternatives (Csibra & Gergely, 1998). However, at this stage agency is understood purely in terms of physical actions and constraints. Infants expect actors to behave rationally, given physically apparent goal states and the physical constraints of the situation (Gergely & Csibra, 2003). The infant does not yet have any idea about the agent's mental state. We have suggested that there is a connection between this focus on understanding actions in terms of their physical as opposed to mental outcomes (a teleological stance) and the mode of experience of agency that we often see in the self-destructive acts of individuals with borderline personality disorder (see below). For these individuals, slight changes in the physical world can trigger elaborate conclusions about states of mind and only modifications in the realm of the physical can convince them as to the intentions of the other.

(b) *During the second year*, children begin to understand that they and others are intentional agents whose actions are caused by prior states of mind, such as desires (Wellman & Phillips, 2001), and that their actions can bring about changes in minds as well as bodies (e.g. by pointing, Corkum & Moore, 1995). At this stage the capacity for emotion regulation comes to reflect the prior and current relationship with the primary caregiver (Calkins & Johnson, 1998). Most importantly, children begin to acquire an internal state language and the ability to reason non-egocentrically about feelings and desires in others (Repacholi & Gopnik, 1997). Paradoxically, this becomes evident not only through the increase in joint goal-directed activity but also through teasing and provocation of younger siblings (Dunn, 1988). However, the child is not yet able to represent mental states independently of physical reality and therefore the distinction between internal and external, appearance and reality is not yet fully achieved (Flavell & Miller, 1998). This means that internal reality is sometimes experienced as far more compelling and at other times seems inconsequential relative to the child's awareness of the physical world. We have referred to these modes of experiencing internal reality as psychic equivalence and pretend modes respectively (see below).

(c) *Around three to four years of age*, the child begins to grasp that people's actions are caused by their beliefs. A meta-analytic review of over 500 tests showed that by and large children younger than three fail the false-belief task (i.e. are unable to attribute a false belief to someone else); as the child's age increases, the child becomes increasingly likely to pass (Wellman *et al.*, 2001), suggesting that mentalizing abilities take a quantum leap forward around age four. From this point, the child can understand both himself and others as representational agents. He knows that people do not always feel what they appear to feel, and that their emotional reactions to an event are influenced by their current mood or even by earlier emotional experiences which were linked to similar events (Flavell & Miller, 1998). Reaching this milestone transforms his social interactions. His understanding of emotions comes to be associated with empathic behaviour (Zahn-Waxler *et al.*, 1992) and more positive peer relations (Dunn & Cutting, 1999). His understanding that human behaviour can be influenced by transient mental states (such as thoughts and feelings) as well as by stable characteristics (such as personality or capability) creates the basis for a structure to underpin an emerging self-concept (Flavell, 1999). His newfound ability to attribute mistaken beliefs to himself and others enriches his repertoire of social interaction: he can now engage in tricks, jokes and deceptions (Sodian & Frith, 1992; Sodian *et al.*, 1992). Notably, the child also begins to prefer playing with peers to playing with adults at this time (Dunn, 1994). This shift brings to a close the time when mentalization was acquired through the agency of an adult mind and opens a lifelong phase of seeking to enhance the capacity to understand self and others in mental state terms through bonds with individuals who share one's interest and humour.

(d) *In the sixth year*, we see related advances, such as the child's ability to relate memories of his intentional activities and experiences into a coherent causal-temporal organization, leading to the establishment of the temporally extended self (Povinelli & Eddy, 1995). Full experience of agency in social interaction can emerge only when actions of the self and other can be understood as initiated and guided by assumptions concerning the emotions, desires and beliefs of both. Further ToM skills that become part of the child's repertoire at this stage include second order ToM (the capacity to understand mistaken beliefs about beliefs), mixed emotions (e.g. understanding being in a conflict), the way expectations or biases might influence the interpretation of ambiguous events, and the capacity for subtle forms of social deceptions (e.g. white lies). As these skills are acquired, the need for physical violence begins to decline (Tremblay, 2000) and relational aggression increases (Cote *et al.*, 2002).

Subjectivity before mentalization

In order to make use of this model of the emergence of mentalizing function in understanding children's subjective experience, we also need a clear conception of what the non-mentalizing mind might be like before the child fully recognizes that his internal states are mere representations of reality. It is important to grasp that, at first, the small child assumes that what he knows is known by others and vice versa. Our sense of the uniqueness of our own perspective develops only slowly. Infants already possess a distinct sense of their physical integrity by approximately three months at the latest, but we start with the assumption that knowledge is common and that our own thoughts or feelings are shared by others. Young children assume that other children will know facts that they themselves have just learnt (Taylor *et al.*, 1994). One reason why toddlers are so prone to outbursts of rage and frustration may be that they expect other people to know what they are thinking and feeling, and to see situations in the same way they do, because the world and individual minds are not yet clearly demarcated. Thus, frustration of their wishes seems malign or wilfully obtuse, rather than the result of a different point of view or alternative priorities.

In describing the normal development of mentalizing in the child of two to five years (Fonagy & Target, 1996; Target & Fonagy, 1996), we have suggested that there is a transition from a split mode of experience to mentalization. We hypothesize that the very young child equates the internal world with the external: what exists in the mind must exist 'out there' and what exists 'out there' must also exist in the mind. At this stage there is no room yet for alternative perspectives: 'How I see it is how it is'. The toddler's or young preschool child's insistence that 'there is a tiger under the bed' is not allayed by parental reassurance. This *psychic equivalence*, as a mode of experiencing the internal world, can cause intense distress, since the experience of a fantasy as potentially real can be terrifying.

At other times, young children appear to be able to use the notion of mental states but paradoxically use it only when they can clearly separate it from physical reality (for example, in play). In this state of mind, which we have called *pretend mode*, thoughts and feelings can be envisioned and talked about but they correspond to nothing real, and are thought to have no implications for the outside world ('pretend mode').

Finally, the compelling nature of physical reality is also obvious when children only impute intention from what is physically apparent. We noted that this *teleological mode* of thinking was present from a very early stage but is compelling for all of us at moments when mentalizing has ceased, when physical reassurance is demanded and required if emotion regulation is to be reinstated.

Normally, at around four years old, the child integrates these modes to arrive at mentalization, in which mental states can be experienced as representations. Inner and outer reality can then be seen as linked, yet differing in important ways, and no longer have to be either equated or dissociated from each other (Gopnik, 1993). However, under certain circumstances, prementalistic forms of subjectivity may still re-emerge to dominate social cognition years after the acquisition of full mentalization.

Mentalizing in families

While on the one hand we have contended that the infant's early relationship to its caregivers is the cradle of mentalizing, on the other hand there is no context more likely to induce a loss of mentalizing than family interactions. It is within the family that relationships tend to be at their most fraught, their most loving, and their most intense emotionally: in other words, the family is an environment with the potential to stimulate a loss of mentalizing in one or more members of the family, on a daily basis. Mentalizing problems may emerge in a variety of contexts and with differing severity and presentations. These occur along a spectrum from relatively mild and specific difficulties to highly destructive non-mentalizing attitudes that may have long-term effects on a child's mentalizing capacity and well-being. Mentalizing strategies may also be under-used or applied erratically because of other demands or high levels of perceived stress, or if a family member or a relationship has a circumscribed 'blind spot'. At the more extreme end of the spectrum, one or more family members may consciously or unconsciously misuse mentalization in their dealings with others.

Sometimes specific problems with mentalizing may occur. For example, in an acrimonious parental separation, one parent, who is otherwise highly sensitive to the child's feeling states, may find it particularly hard to tune into the child's feelings and thoughts about the loss of the parental couple, perhaps because of ongoing hatred of the other parent. As a result the parent is unable to mentalize that aspect of his or her child's life.

A specific loss of mentalization such as this may be associated with stress: when exposed to great pressure, most people tend to lose their capacity to think about the thoughts and feelings of others. For example, quite dramatic temporary failures of mentalization can arise in individuals and families during emotionally intense interchanges. This can also happen merely in response to thoughts and feelings that trigger high arousal and anti-mentalizing reactions. Under such circumstances, grossly inaccurate or even seemingly malevolent feelings can be attributed to others and feelings of resentment and mistrust grow in the relationship context. The representation of the mind of others can literally be obliterated and replaced by an empty or hostile image. For example, when a parent becomes convinced that their child is deliberately and maliciously provoking them, his or her mind becomes closed to seeing the child in alternative ways. Or a parent who suffered physical or sexual abuse may temporarily lose the capacity to mentalize, when faced with a reminder of their own (past) states of helplessness, anger or shame. Their child's distressed response may act as an additional reminder.

In other situations a parent may be temporarily preoccupied with other important concrete issues in their life, such as a crisis at work, and this may propel them into a non-mentalizing frame that gets carried into the family life. This state may fluctuate, preventing the parent from being attuned to the child's feeling states at certain times. In such a scenario, the child, who usually has had good experiences of feeling thought about and understood, is suddenly confused by the parent's apparent emotional unavailability. The problem can be compounded further if the parent is incapable of appreciating the child's disappointment and confusion. Other specific family problems with mentalizing can arise from the child obscuring his or her own mental states, making the parent's task of 'mind-reading' difficult. This can happen for a wide range of reasons, such as the arrival of a new step-parent, or in the course of limited visitation rights, when the non-resident parent simply lacks the contextual information necessary to make sense of the child's state of mind. In both these cases, the parent's understandable inability to mentalize the child can nevertheless leave the child feeling that they are not understood, limiting their motivation for making themselves available to be understood.

There are background conditions that increase the frequency with which non-mentalizing family interactions arise. Longstanding mental heath problems can compromise mentalizing in families in a number of ways. A parent with schizophrenia, particularly with repeated episodes of the illness, may find it difficult to take alternative perspectives into account, to develop and model a trusting attitude, or to take turns, and may also have strong unshakable beliefs which will impede curiosity and reflective contemplation. A child in such a family may respond to this from early on by 'hyper-mentalizing' – being a precocious mentalizer – as part of his or her development into a 'young carer'. Other children appear to disengage from the mental state of adults. In both scenarios, an interest in the child's own mental state decreases as a consequence of the parents' impaired mentalizing.

Where a parent suffers from major depression, the child may be overactive in stimulating the parent, not into a mentalizing attitude but rather into action in order to break through oppositional behaviours as ways of making the parent connect, even if only via disciplining and other non-mentalizing actions. Some children may adopt a stance analogous to that of their parents, shutting down and opting for not thinking as the least painful way of coping with emotional neglect. Parents with high levels of arousal, such as those with chronic anxiety states, can find themselves excessively engaged with the child's mental world, anxiously loading the child with their own anxious preoccupations. The child, who does not understand the source of severe anxiety, can be perturbed by it and search for an explanation in their actions and thoughts, engaging in turn in excessive mentalizing. In a sense, similar processes appear to take place in the parent and child, almost in parallel, but failing to inform each other directly.

When these dyadic processes take place in a family context, it is inevitable that it will affect everyone, with others attempting to mentalize the relationship in question. Another family member, faced with a dyadic non-mentalizing interaction and attempting to understand the two parties, will run the risk of being only partially understood by one or both parties. Each non-mentalizing person is likely to understand only some aspects of the onlooker's stance: those which correspond to their own perspective. At the same time, each person in the dyad will feel invalidated by those aspects of the onlooker's stance which describe the mind state of the other, as though the onlooker has taken sides in opposition to him or her. In that way the onlooker is recruited to the non-mentalizing interaction as they themselves feel that they have only partially been heard by each of the protagonists. In this way, a non-mentalizing dyad becomes a triad. Gradually, the system can recruit other members of the family as well as professionals.

Another systemic perspective on mentalization failure is the experience of the individual faced with non-responsive minds. When faced with family members who cannot respond to a member's enquiring or curious mind, the person will give up, reinforcing the hopelessness of all concerned, resulting in a 'circular' or cyclic hopelessness. For example, a child who is depressed may experience her thoughts and feelings about herself as entirely real, and will be deprived of the perspective that would allow her to think differently about herself or others, as a result of the lack of interest in her state of mind that she experiences from her carers. In the absence of relational mentalizing strengths, such as curiosity or reflective contemplation and perspective taking, pessimism about the possibility of feelings changing takes over. When the child experiences feelings of hopelessness, she immediately takes them to be a 'physical reality' and cannot treat them as 'just a thought' which could then be challenged cognitively. The parents of a depressed child or adolescent may resonate with their child's predicament because they agree with the child's interpretation of her situation (e.g. they all may feel that having few friends is a hopeless situation) or because the child's behaviour may be experienced by them as an expression of their own failure or incompetence. Just as mentalizing engenders more mentalizing, so non-mentalizing can engender further non-mentalizing in a family context.

In families with poor boundaries between the generations (often described as enmeshed – e.g. Minuchin, 1974) forms of intrusive mentalizing can take place. Here the separateness of minds is not respected within the family: a family member strongly believes she or he knows what another member thinks and feels. In such cases, the family discourse may sound as if everyone is mentalizing well, but, paradoxically, this does not have the usual consequence of people feeling understood. We have described such interactions, which are marked by their 'pretend' quality, as pseudo-mentalization. Family members' narratives fail to connect with each other, which may incite each family member to redouble his or her efforts to have his or her view accepted by the rest of the family. In consequence, more and more unjustified assumptions are made about other people's mental states: family members invest a lot of energy in thinking or talking about how other family members think or feel, but their interpretations bear little or no relationship to other people's reality. The result is that mentalization is experienced as being obstructive and confusing and it can lead to certain members of the family avoiding further mentalization efforts altogether.

If a member of the family 'leaves the field', becoming unavailable for mentalizing within the family system, other family members may respond in kind, demonstrating more extreme non-mentalizing by taking on a stance that directly attacks mentalization. Statements indicating this kind of extreme non-mentalizing could include: 'You are trying to drive me crazy'; 'Your grandma is in league with your father against us'; 'You provoked me'; 'You don't care about whether your dad is here or not'; 'You don't care about me'; 'You would be glad if I was dead'. Such statements generate further arousal that is incompatible with mentalization and can lead to nothing but further non-mentalizing cycles. Any attempts to discuss the meaning of such statements are almost certain to fail, as such statements only make sense in a non-mentalizing world. A therapist who attempts to question the meaning of such statements is therefore inadvertently contributing to the non-mentalizing cycle and will at best achieve pseudo-mentalization.

At the extreme end of the non-mentalizing spectrum is the misuse of mentalization. Here, understanding of mental states of self and others is not directly impaired, but is misused to further an individual's interest at the expense of the well-being of the family or one of its members. For example, a parent might use a child's current mental state (e.g. sadness) as ammunition in a marital battle (e.g. 'Whenever you visit your father you feel so sad afterwards, don't you think you should stop seeing him?'). In these situations the child might experience mentalization as aversive because being understood occurs in the context of being manipulated. In such cases, children's feelings are typically exaggerated or distorted in the interest of the parent's unspoken intention or attitude. Another example might be a father who claims that he objects to his wife working because it makes the children feel neglected, whereas the true cause of his objection is that his wife's work requires him to be more involved at home, leaving him less time for himself.

Another misuse of mentalization is coercion against the child's thoughts. This involves the parent undermining the child's capacity to think by deliberately humiliating the child for her or his thoughts and feelings. For example, the parent exposes the child's sexual feelings in a family gathering in a belittling and insensitive manner, disclosing what the child might have confided in private. These phenomena are most pernicious in the context of abuse, where the abusive party may falsely maintain that the child 'fell down the stairs, I never hit you' or that the child 'enjoyed it when I touched you like that', for instance. This kind of misuse of mentalization may undermine the child's capacity to mentalize, not simply because they directly contradict the child's own reality, but because the child may be unable to construct a bearable image of the thoughts that the parent must have had in order to make such confusing statements.

Conclusion

In this chapter we have briefly summarized the relationship between attachment and mentalizing, suggesting that the process of mentalizing should be given central importance in child development. We suggest that a link between abnormal development of social cognition during childhood and adult psychopathology may be partially mediated through mentalizing. This suggestion implies that a focus on mentalizing process could enhance clinical practice – not only with adults, but also clinical practice with children and families. Unlike other integrative approaches, such as interpersonal psychotherapy, mentalization-based treatment has a theoretical frame of reference which includes a developmental model, a theory of psychopathology and a hypothesis about the mechanism of therapeutic action. We suggest that a focus on enhancing mentalizing may be an important factor distinguishing mentalizing therapies from other psychotherapies. The therapist is focused on mental processes and is not engaged in cognitive restructuring, he is not working to provide insight and he does not attempt to alter behaviour directly. The cognitive and behavioural changes that often take place as patients come to recognize underlying meanings or identify reasons why they are as they are occur in MBT as consequences of the change in mentalizing, rather like positive side effects.

Mentalizing could be seen as one of many common factors in psychotherapy. All psychotherapies, whatever their focus, share the potential to recreate an interactional matrix of attachment in which mentalization develops and sometimes flourishes. This perhaps acts as a catalyst for further change in cognitions, emotions and behaviour, irrespective of the therapeutic target. Having a patient's mind in mind will make any therapeutic effort more efficient.

Mentalizing is a developmental construct. This raises questions about the variability not simply of mother–child interaction but of families and the significance of developmental milestones, particularly the importance of the move from childhood to adolescence. Distortions in the development of mentalizing are therefore likely to go beyond the diagnostic group of individuals with personality disorder and there may be other individuals who can benefit from having their mentalizing problems addressed directly. This opens up the possibility of preventive work during childhood. As mentalizing is a fundamental psychological process and so interfaces with all major mental disorders, mentalizing-focused approaches may have the potential to improve well-being across a range of disorders. So, whilst on the one hand our claims for mentalizing continue to be modest, on the other hand, we see it as a unifying mental process that interfaces with, and can therefore interfere with, a wide range of psychological functions. This suggests that, regardless of the approach focusing on mentalizing being adopted in a treatment, there is a need for any practitioner to see the world from the patient's perspective. For all clinicians, there is an intrinsic value in maintaining a focus on the patient's internal mental process because this demonstrates a powerful commitment to the patient's subjectivity.

References

Ainsworth, M. D. S., Blehar, M. C., Waters, E., & Wall, S. (1978). *Patterns of attachment: A psychological study of the strange situation*. Hillsdale, NJ: Lawrence Erlbaum Associates, Inc.

Allen, J., Fonagy, P., & Bateman, A. (2008). *Mentalizing in clinical practice*. Washington, DC: American Psychiatric Press.

Bahrick, L. R., & Watson, J. S. (1985). Detection of intermodal proprioceptive-visual contingency as a potential basis of self-perception in infancy. *Developmental Psychology*, 21, 963–973.

Baldwin, D. A., Baird, J. A., Saylor, M. M., & Clark, M. A. (2001). Infants parse dynamic action. *Child Development*, 72(3), 708–717.

Bowlby, J. (1969). *Attachment and Loss, Vol. 1: Attachment*. London: Hogarth Press and the Institute of Psycho-Analysis.

Bowlby, J. (1973). *Attachment and Loss, Vol. 2: Separation: Anxiety and anger*. London: Hogarth Press and Institute of Psycho-Analysis.

Bronfman, E., Parsons, E., & Lyons-Ruth, K. (1999). Atypical Maternal Behavior Instrument for Assessment and Classification (AMBIANCE): Manual for coding disrupted affective communication, version 2. Unpublished manuscript. Cambridge, MA: Harvard Medical School.

Calkins, S., & Johnson, M. (1998). Toddler regulation of distress to frustrating events: Temperamental and maternal correlates. *Infant Behavior and Development*, 21, 379–395.

Cicchetti, D., Rogosch, F. A., Maughan, A., Toth, S. L., & Bruce, J. (2003). False belief understanding in maltreated children. *Developmental Psychopathology*, 15(4), 1067–1091.

Cicchetti, D., & Valentino, K. (2006). An ecological-transactional perspective on child maltreatment: Failure of the average expectable environment and its influence on child development. In D. Cicchetti & D. J. Cohen (Eds.), *Developmental psychopathology*. (2nd ed., Vol. 3, pp. 129–201). New York: Wiley.

Corkum, V., & Moore, C. (1995). Development of joint visual attention in infants. In C. Moore & P. Dunham (Eds.), *Joint attention: Its origins and role in development* (pp. 61–83). New York: Lawrence Erlbaum Associates, Inc.

Cote, S., Tremblay, R. E., Nagin, D., Zoccolillo, M., & Vitaro, F. (2002). The development of impulsivity, fearfulness, and helpfulness during childhood: Patterns of consistency and change in the trajectories of boys and girls. *Journal of Child Psychology and Psychiatry and Allied Disciplines*, 43(5), 609–618.

Crittenden, P. M. (1990). Internal representational models of attachment relationships. *Infant Mental Health Journal*, 11, 259–277.

Csibra, G., & Gergely, G. (1998). The teleological origins of mentalistic action explanations: A developmental hypothesis. *Developmental Science*, 1(2), 255–259.

Dunn, J. (1988). *The beginnings of social understanding*. Oxford: Blackwell and Cambridge, MA: Harvard University Press.

Dunn, J. (1994). Changing minds and changing relationships. In C. Lewis & P. Mitchell (Eds.), *Children's early understanding of mind: Origins and development* (pp. 297–310). Hove, UK: Lawrence Erlbaum Associates, Inc.

Dunn, J., & Cutting, A. L. (1999). Understanding others, and individual differences in friendship interactions in young children. *Social Development*, 8(2), 202–219.

Fearon, R. M., Van Ijzendoorn, M. H., Fonagy, P., Bakermans-Kranenburg, M. J., Schuengel, C., & Bokhorst, C. L. (2006). In search of shared and nonshared environmental factors in security of attachment: A behavior-genetic study of the association between sensitivity and attachment security. *Developmental Psychology*, 42(6), 1026–1040.

Flavell, J. H. (1999). Cognitive development: Children's knowledge about the mind. *Annual Review of Psychology*, 50, 21–45.

Flavell, J. H., & Miller, P. H. (1998). Social cognition. In W. Damon, D. Kuhn & R. S. Siegler (Eds.), *Handbook of child psychology* (5th ed., pp. 851–898). New York: Wiley.

Fonagy, P. (1989). On tolerating mental states: Theory of mind in borderline patients. *Bulletin of the Anna Freud Centre*, 12, 91–115.

Fonagy, P. (1991). Thinking about thinking: Some clinical and theoretical considerations in the treatment of a borderline patient. *International Journal of Psycho-Analysis*, 72, 1–18.

Fonagy, P., & Higgitt, A. (1989). A developmental perspective on borderline personality disorder. *Revue Internationale de Psychopathologie*, 1, 125–159.

Fonagy, P., & Luyten, P. (2009). A developmental, mentalization-based approach to the understanding and treatment of borderline personality disorder. *Development and Psychopathology*, 21(4), 1355–1381.

Fonagy, P., & Target, M. (1996). Playing with reality: I. Theory of mind and the normal development of psychic reality. *International Journal of Psycho-Analysis*, 77, 217–233.

Fonagy, P., & Target, M. (2000). Playing with reality III: The persistence of dual psychic reality in borderline patients. *International Journal of Psychoanalysis*, 81(5), 853–874.

Fonagy, P., & Target, M. (2007). Playing with reality: IV. A theory of external reality rooted in intersubjectivity. *International Journal of Psychoanalysis*, 88(Pt 4), 917–937.

Fonagy, P., Steele, H., & Steele, M. (1991a). Maternal representations of attachment during pregnancy predict the organization of infant–mother attachment at one year of age. *Child Development*, 62, 891–905.

Fonagy, P., Steele, M., Moran, G. S., Steele, H., & Higgitt, A. C. (1991b). Measuring the ghost in the nursery: a summary of the main findings of the Anna Freud Centre/University College London parent–child study. *Bulletin of the Anna Freud Centre*, 14, 115–131.

Fonagy, P., Redfern, S., & Charman, T. (1997a). The relationship between belief–desire reasoning and a projective measure of attachment security (SAT). *British Journal of Developmental Psychology*, 15, 51–61.

Fonagy, P., Steele, M., Steele, H., & Target, M. (1997b). *Reflective-functioning manual, version 4.1, for application to adult attachment interviews*. London: University College London.

Fonagy, P., Gergely, G., Jurist, E., & Target, M. (2002). *Affect regulation, mentalization and the development of the self*. New York: Other Press.

Fraiberg, S. (1977). *Insights from the blind*. London: Souvenir Press.

Freud, A. (1936). *The ego and the mechanisms of defence*. New York: International Universities Press, 1946.

Frodi, A., & Smetana, J. (1984). Abused, neglected, and nonmaltreated preschoolers' ability to discriminate emotions in others: The effects of IQ. *Child Abuse & Neglect*, 8(4), 459–465.

George, C., & Solomon, J. (1999). A comparison of attachment theory and psychoanalytic approaches to mothering. *Psychoanalytic Inquiry*, 19, 618–646.

George, C., Kaplan, N., & Main, M. (1985). The Adult Attachment Interview. Unpublished manuscript, Department of Psychology, University of California at Berkeley.

Gergely, G. (2001). The obscure object of desire: 'Nearly, but clearly not, like me'. Contingency preference in normal children versus children with autism. In J. Allen, P. Fonagy & G. Gergely (Eds.), *Contingency perception and attachment in infancy, special issue of the Bulletin of the Menninger Clinic* (pp. 411–426). New York: Guilford Press.

Gergely, G., & Csibra, G. (2003). Teleological reasoning in infancy: The naive theory of rational action. *Trends in Cognitive Sciences*, 7, 287–292.

Gergely, G., & Watson, J. (1996). The social biofeedback model of parental affect-mirroring. *International Journal of Psycho-Analysis*, 77, 1181–1212.

Gergely, G., & Watson, J. (1999). Early social-emotional development: Contingency perception and the social biofeedback model. In P. Rochat (Ed.), *Early social cognition: Understanding others in the first months of life* (pp. 101–137). Hillsdale, NJ: Lawrence Erlbaum Associates, Inc.

Gopnik, A. (1993). How we know our minds: The illusion of first-person knowledge of intentionality. *Behavioral and Brain Sciences*, 16, 1–14, 29–113.

Grienenberger, J. F., Kelly, K., & Slade, A. (2005). Maternal reflective functioning, mother–infant affective communication, and infant attachment: Exploring the link between mental states and observed caregiving behavior in the intergenerational transmission of attachment. *Attachment & Human Development*, 7(3), 299–311.

Hill, J., Fonagy, P., Safier, E., & Sargent, J. (2003). The ecology of attachment in the family. *Family Process*, 42(2), 205–221.

Hobson, R. P., & Bishop, M. (2003). The pathogenesis of autism: Insights from congenital blindness. *Philosophical Transactions of the Royal Society London B Bioogical Sciences*, 358(1430), 335–344.

Hofer, M. A. (1995). Hidden regulators: Implications for a new understanding of attachment, separation and loss. In S. Goldberg, R. Muir & J. Kerr (Eds.), *Attachment theory: Social, developmental, and clinical perspectives* (pp. 203–230). Hillsdale, NJ: Analytic Press.

Hofer, M. A. (2004). The emerging neurobiology of attachment and separation: How parents shape their infant's brain and behavior. In S. W. Coates & J. L. Rosenthal (Eds.), *September 11 – 'When the bough broke', attachment theory, psychobiology, and social policy: An integrated approach to trauma*. New York: Analytic Press.

Legerstee, M., & Varghese, J. (2001). The role of maternal affect mirroring on social expectancies in 2–3 month-old infants. *Child Development*, 72, 1301–1313.

Leslie, A. M. (1987). Pretense and representation: The origins of 'Theory of Mind'. *Psychological Review*, 94, 412–426.

Leslie, A. M. (1994). TOMM, ToBy, and agency: Core architecture and domain specificity. In L. Hirschfeld & S. Gelman (Eds.), *Mapping the mind: Domain specificity in cognition and culture* (pp. 119–148). New York: Cambridge University Press.

Lewis, V., Norgate, S., Collis, G., & Reynolds, R. (2000). The consequences of visual impairment for children's symbolic and functional play. *British Journal of Developmental Psychology*, 18, 449–464.

Lieberman, M. (2007). Social cognitive neuroscience: A review of core processes. *Annual Review of Psychology*, 58, 259–289.

Luyten, P., Fonagy, P., Mayes, L., Vermote, R., Lowyck, B., Bateman, A., *et al.* (submitted). Broadening the scope of the mentalization-based approach to psychopathology.

Lyons-Ruth, K., & Jacobvitz, D. (2008). Attachment disorganization: Unresolved loss, relational violence, and lapses in behavioral and attentional strategies. In J. Cassidy & P. R. Shaver (Eds.), *Handbook of attachment: Theory, research and clinical applications* (pp. 520–554). New York: Guilford Press.

McAlpine, L. M., & Moore, C. L. (1985). The development of social understanding in children with visual impairments. *Journal of Visual Impairment and Blindness*, 89, 349–358.

Main, M. (1997). Attachment narratives and attachment across the lifespan. Paper presented at the Fall Meeting of the American Psychoanalytic Association, New York.

Main, M., & Hesse, E. (2000). The organized categories of infant, child, and adult attachment: Flexible vs. inflexible attention under attachment-related stress. *Journal of the American Psychoanalytic Association*, 48, 1055–1096.

Meins, E., Ferryhough, C., Fradley, E., & Tuckey, M. (2001). Rethinking maternal sensitivity: Mothers' comments on infants' mental processes predict security of attachment at 12 months. *Journal of Child Psychology and Psychiatry*, 42, 637–648.

Minuchin, S. (1974). *Families and family therapy*. Cambridge, MA: Harvard University Press.

Mitchell, R. W. (1993). Mental models of mirror self-recognition: Two theories. *New Ideas in Psychology*, 11, 295–325.

Neisser, U. (1988). Five kinds of self-knowledge. *Philosophical Psychology*, 1, 35–59.

Newton, P., Reddy, V., & Bull, R. (2000). Children's everyday deception and performance on false-belief tasks. *British Journal of Developmental Psychology*, 18, 297–317.

Oppenheim, D., & Koren-Karie, N. (2002). Mothers' insightfulness regarding their children's internal worlds: The capacity underlying secure child–mother relationships. *Infant Mental Health Journal*, 23, 593–605.

Pears, K. C., & Fisher, P. A. (2005). Emotion understanding and theory of mind among maltreated children in foster care. *Development and Psychopathology*, 17(1), 47–65.

Pears, K. C., & Moses, L. J. (2003). Demographics, parenting, and theory of mind in preschool children. *Social Development*, 12, 1–20.

Povinelli, D. J., & Eddy, T. J. (1995). The unduplicated self. In P. Rochat (Ed.), *The self in infancy: Theory and research* (pp. 161–192). Amsterdam: Elsevier.

Repacholi, B. M., & Gopnik, A. (1997). Early reasoning about desires: Evidence from 14- and 18-month-olds. *Developmental Psychology*, 33, 12–21.

Rosenfeld, H. (1971). Contribution to the psychopathology of psychotic states: The importance of projective identification in the ego structure and object relations of the psychotic patient. In E. B. Spillius (Ed.), *Melanie Klein today* (pp. 117–137). London: Routledge, 1988.

Saxe, R. (2006). Uniquely human social cognition. *Current Opinion Neurobiology*, 16(2), 235–239.

Sharp, C., Fonagy, P., & Goodyer, I. (2006). Imagining your child's mind: Psychosocial adjustment and mothers' ability to predict their children's attributional response styles. *British Journal of Developmental Psychology*, 24(1), 197–214.

Siegal, M., & Patterson, C. C. (2008). Language and theory of mind in atypically developing children: Evidence from studies of deafness, blindness, and autism. In C. Sharp, P. Fonagy & I. Goodyer (Eds.), *Social cognition and developmental psychology*. Oxford: Oxford University Press.

Slade, A., Grienenberger, J., Bernbach, E., Levy, D., & Locker, A. (2005). Maternal reflective functioning, attachment and the transmission gap: A preliminary study. *Attachment and Human Development*, 7(3), 283–298.

Smith, M., & Walden, T. (1999). Understanding feelings and coping with emotional situations: A comparison of maltreated and nonmaltreated preschoolers. *Social Development*, 8(1), 93–116.

Sodian, B., & Frith, U. (1992). Deception and sabotage in autistic, retarded and normal children. *Journal of Child Psychology and Psychiatry*, 33(3), 591–605.

Sodian, B., Taylor, C., Harris, P. L., & Perner, J. (1992). Early deception and the child's theory of mind: False trails and genuine markers. *Child Development*, 62, 468–483.

Sroufe, L. A. (1996). *Emotional development: The organization of emotional life in the early years*. New York: Cambridge University Press.

Steele, H., Steele, M., & Fonagy, P. (unpublished manuscript). A path-analytic model of determinants of infant–parent attachment: Limited rather than multiple pathways.

Target, M., & Fonagy, P. (1996). Playing with reality II: The development of psychic reality from a theoretical perspective. *International Journal of Psycho-Analysis*, 77, 459–479.

Taylor, M., Esbensen, B. M., & Bennett, R. T. (1994). Children's understanding of knowledge acquisition: The tendency for children to report that they have always known what they have just learned. *Child Development*, 65(6), 1581–1604.

Tremblay, R. E. (2000). The origins of youth violence. *ISUMA*, Autumn, 19–24.

van IJzendoorn, M. H. (1995). Adult attachment representations, parental responsiveness, and infant attachment: A meta-analysis on the predictive validity of the Adult Attachment Interview. *Psychological Bulletin*, 117, 387–403.

Watson, J. S. (1994). Detection of self: The perfect algorithm. In S. Parker, R. Mitchell & M. Boccia (Eds.), *Self-Awareness in animals and humans: Developmental perspectives* (pp. 131–149) Cambridge: Cambridge University Press.

Wellman, H. M., Cross, D., & Watson, J. (2001). Meta-analysis of theory-of-mind development: The truth about false belief. *Child Development*, 72(3), 655–684.

Wellman, H. M., & Phillips, A. T. (2001). Developing intentional understandings. In L. Moses, B. Male & D. Baldwin (Eds.), *Intentionality: A key to human understanding*. Cambridge, MA: MIT Press.

Winnicott, D. W. (1965). Ego distortion in terms of true and false self. In *The maturational process and the facilitating environment* (pp. 140–152). New York: International Universities Press.

Zahn-Waxler, C., Radke-Yarrow, M., Wagner, E., & Chapman, M. (1992). Development of concern for others. *Developmental Psychology*, 28, 126–136.

Chapter 2

Mentalizing problems in children and adolescents

Carla Sharp and Amanda Venta

A taxonomy for mentalizing failures in children and adolescents

Imagine a movie scene that starts with the doorbell ringing. A young and attractive woman named Sandra opens the front door. Upon opening the door, a man, who looks to be around the same age as Sandra, enters the house. Sandra says 'Hi' and the man asks her whether she is surprised. Before she can answer, he tells her that she looks terrific. He asks whether she did something with her hair. Sandra touches her hair and starts to say something but the young man interrupts, telling her that her hair looks very classy. The movie then stops and you are asked to answer the following question: 'What is Sandra feeling? (1) that her hair does not look nice; (2) that she is pleased about his compliment; (3) that she is exasperated about the man coming on too strong; or (4) that she is flattered but somewhat taken by surprise?'

The above movie scene is the first scene of an exciting new approach to measuring mentalizing in research studies. The measure, named the Movie for the Assessment of Social Cognition (MASC; Dziobek *et al.*, 2006), asks individuals to watch a 15-minute film about four characters (Sandra, Michael, Betty and Cliff) getting together for a dinner party. The characters in the film display stable characteristics (traits) that are different from one another (e.g. outgoing, timid, selfish, etc.). Themes of each segment cover friendship and dating issues, so that each character experiences different situations through the course of the film. These situations are meant to elicit emotions and mental states such as anger, affection, gratefulness, jealousy, fear, ambition, embarrassment, or disgust. The relationships between the characters vary in the amount of intimacy (friends to strangers) and thus represent different social reference systems on which mental state inferences have to be made.

Of course, readers of the current chapter did not have the benefit of seeing the facial expressions of the two characters in the movie clip described above, but if a reader guessed the correct answer to be (4), that she is flattered but somewhat taken by surprise, then this reader can consider herself a good and accurate mentalizer. According to the MASC developers, the other three categories of mentalizing include no theory of mind or *no mentalizing* (Sandra felt that her hair does not look nice); less theory of mind or *under-mentalizing* (Sandra felt pleased about his compliment) and excessive theory of mind or *hyper-mentalizing* (Sandra felt exasperated about the man coming on too strong). We may add to this list the concepts of *distorted mentalizing* (Sharp, 2006) and *pseudo-mentalizing* (Allen *et al.*, 2008). We will return to definitions of each type of mentalizing failure later in the chapter, but briefly, distorted mentalizing refers to mind *mis*reading (Allen, 2006) or biased mindreading (Sharp *et al.*, 2007) where mental states are attributed to other minds, but in a systematically biased way. Pseudo-mentalizing refers to mindreading that looks like mentalizing, but lacks some of the essential features of genuine mentalizing (Allen *et al.*, 2008).

It is clear from the example above that, beyond a complete lack of mentalizing, there are multiple ways in which mentalizing can go awry – collectively (and in jest) referred to by Allen *et al.* (2008: 30) as '*excrementalizing*: mentalizing, but doing a crappy job of it'. In this chapter, we will review mentalizing problems in children and adolescents using the taxonomy outlined above. Our goal is thereby: (1) to establish mentalizing as an important endophenotype to be targeted in treatment; and (2) to illuminate how different aspects of mentalizing are reflected in the heterogeneity of different childhood disorders. Taken together, the current chapter will emphasize the importance of targeting and measuring change in treatment via mentalizing failures across divergent childhood and adolescent disorders.

No mentalizing: Are autistic individuals mindblind?

The term mentalizing is often used interchangeably with the concept of theory of mind (ToM). The ToM framework has been associated with one of the fastest growing bodies of empirical research in psychology over the last 30 years (Leudar & Costall, 2010), and it is within this framework that the notion of 'no mentalizing' underlying autistic spectrum disorders (ASDs) has been investigated. Most researchers in this area take a cognitive modularist view of mentalizing, akin to Chomsky's (1980) conceptualization of language development as a set of linguistic schemata that are hard-wired in the structure of the human brain. At its most extreme, modularist researchers view autism as an example of a clinical condition where the ToM module has been excised as though by a lesion (Belmonte, 2008).

The first evidence for the notion that autistic individuals may lack a ToM module was provided in a now much-cited study by Baron-Cohen *et al.* (1985). A group of 11-year-old autistic children was compared with age-matched children with Down's syndrome and four-year-old clinically normal children on a 'false belief' task. During the task, a doll character (Sally) placed an object in a basket. Then, another character (Anne) hid the object in a different location while Sally was out of the room. Participants were asked where Sally would look for the object on return. Results indicated that, despite the fact that the mental age of the autistic children was higher than that of the Down's syndrome and normal controls, 80 per cent of the autistic children were unable to demonstrate an understanding of Sally's false belief regarding the object's location, while the majority of Down's syndrome and normal subjects did. The authors concluded that autistic children may lack the capacity to build theories on the content (beliefs or false beliefs) of others' minds – a deficit famously coined 'mind-blindness' (Baron-Cohen, 1995).

Under-mentalizing: not enough of a good thing

Despite initial evidence for a complete lack of ToM associated with autism, evidence also appeared indicating that a significant number of autistic children and adolescents passed false belief tasks (Frith & Happé, 1994). Moreover, many ToM researchers started reformulating the concept within a continuum of variation, as opposed to viewing it categorically. For instance, Baron-Cohen and colleagues (Baron-Cohen *et al.*, 2003; Baron-Cohen & Wheelright, 2004) developed an approach to mentalizing where ToM became a lower level module of a broader continuum of 'empathizing' capacity. In this approach, autistic children can be situated on an empathizing continuum, albeit at its lower extreme.

Further expanding the continuum view of ToM was a growing literature demonstrating impairments in even lower level modules preceding the development of ToM subsumed under the broad continuum of empathizing. For instance, autistic infants have demonstrated a general lack of social interest, reduced levels of social engagement and social-communicative exchanges, limited eye contact and less visual attention to social stimuli (Volkmar *et al.*, 2005). Moreover, reduced mentalizing continued through the toddler years in autistic children. Two-year-olds with autism were shown to be more limited in imitation, pretend play and symbolic representation of a shared object (Charman & Baron-Cohen, 1997; Charman *et al.*, 1997; Roeyers *et al.*, 1998) – a limitation that was demonstrated even for older children with autism (Hobson & Lee, 1999; Loveland & Tunali, 1994; Smith & Bryson, 1994). These children are less likely to make mental-physical or appearance-reality distinctions, and are less likely to understand the functions of the brain or mind (Baron-Cohen, 1989). They perform less well on 'seeing-leads-to-knowing' tests[1] (Baron-Cohen & Goodhart, 1994) and

1 'Seeing-leads-to-knowing' or 'see-know' tests assess children's understanding that visual access to information is a way of gaining knowledge of that information (Wimmer *et al.*, 1988). In a typical 'seeing-leads-to-knowing' task, participants are given a story about two characters, and are required to ascribe knowledge or ignorance of the contents of an opaque box to characters who either have or have not looked inside the box.

are worse at distinguishing mental from non-mental verbs (Baron-Cohen *et al.*, 1994). They exhibit less spontaneous pretend play (Baron-Cohen, 1987), display difficulties in understanding complex mental states (Baron-Cohen, 1991), have trouble following gaze direction (Leekam & Perner, 1991), have reduced insight into deception (Yirmiya & Shulman, 1996), and tend to conflate memories of their own actions with memories of the actions of other people (Russell & Jarrold, 1999). Taken together, a solid body of literature suggests reduced mentalizing capacity in autistic children and adolescents across all developmental stages. Consequently, a range of interventions has been developed with the shared goal of increasing communication and joint social interaction in autistic children with positive results (Aldred *et al.*, 2004; Howlin *et al.*, 2007; Kasari *et al.*, 2006).

To mentalize or not to mentalize: hyper-mentalizing and under-mentalizing in schizophrenia

The negative symptom cluster of early-onset schizophrenia in adolescence seems to show a similar pattern of reduced mentalizing, as observed in autism (Tordjman, 2008). Impairments in tests of recognizing expression from eyes and faces have been identified in schizophrenia, similar to autism (e.g. Kington *et al.*, 2000). However, these mentalization failures appear to be a function of inaccurate inferences of mental states from gaze associated with the positive symptoms of schizophrenia, rather than the underdevelopment or absence of mental-state attribution ascribed to autistic cognition (Langdon & Brock, 2008). Langdon and colleagues interpret the paranoid features of some of the positive symptoms of psychosis (such as delusions) as forms of hyper-mentalizing, such that ToM is dysregulated via impaired, inflexible, or extreme inferences regarding social cues and over-attribution of mental states and intentions (Harrington *et al.*, 2005; Langdon *et al.*, 2006). Put simply, according to this view, people with schizophrenia tend to ascribe intentions where none exist.

The curious mixture of under and hyper-mentalizing in schizophrenia was further demonstrated by Langdon (2005) in a study where individuals with schizophrenia were presented with ToM cartoons that required accurate mental-state inferences in order to understand a joke vs. a non-mentalistic control condition. People with schizophrenia used less mental-state language than healthy controls in the mentalistic conditions, but inappropriately ascribed mental states to characters in the non-mentalistic condition. Langdon and colleagues (Langdon, 2003; Langdon & Coltheart, 2001; Langdon *et al.*, 2001) explained hyper-mentalizing as born from the inability to take perspectives. In essence, individuals with schizophrenia find it hard to mindread (under-mentalizing) and consequently project their own paranoid suspicions and biases onto others (hyper-mentalizing).

Hyper-mentalizing: too much of a good thing

In describing the tendency to hyper-mentalize in individuals with schizophrenia, Langdon and Brock (2008) quote Nesse (2004: 62) in writing that 'those who have worked with schizophrenics know the eerie feeling of being with someone whose intuitions are acutely tuned to the subtlest unintentional cues, even while the person is incapable of accurate empathic understanding'. This statement may very well have been written by clinicians who work with borderline personality disorder (BPD). Indeed, the BPD 'paradox' of apparently impaired interpersonal functioning and enhanced emotional sensitivity was described even before the explosion of mentalizing research in this area (Krohn, 1974).

In a recent study (Sharp *et al.*, 2011), we used the task described in the opening paragraphs of this chapter to investigate, for the first time, mentalizing problems in adolescents with borderline traits. While other studies have investigated aspects of emotional processing in borderline youth (von Ceumern-Lindenstjerna *et al.*, 2010), ours was the first to use a ToM task that resembled the demands of everyday social cognition. It was also the first to assess mentalizing impairment in BPD specifically by considering potential dysfunctions of mentalizing such as hyper-mentalizing, which results in incorrect, 'reduced' mental state attribution as opposed to a complete lack of ToM. Results of this study showed that neither under-mentalizing nor the complete absence of mentalizing was linked to borderline traits in adolescents. Rather, hyper-mentalizing (over-interpretive mental state reasoning) was strongly associated with BPD features in adolescents. Those with BPD features showed a tendency to make overly complex inferences based on social cues, which resulted in errors. Thus, they tended to over-interpret social signs. These results stand in contrast to studies using this task in other psychiatric populations which identify general difficulties in ToM in individuals with autistic spectrum disorders (ASDs; Dziobek *et al.*, 2006) and under-mentalizing in adults with euthymic bipolar disorder (Montag *et al.*, 2009). Although internalizing and externalizing symptoms as well as female sex were also associated with hyper-mentalizing in our study, controlling for these did not eliminate the prediction of borderline traits from hyper-mentalizing. Moreover, follow-up analyses demonstrated a mediating effect for difficulties in emotion regulation in the relation between hyper-mentalizing and borderline traits.

Taken together, the results from this study confirm clinical (Allen, 2002; Bateman & Fonagy, 2004) and theoretical (Sharp & Fonagy, 2008b) evidence that in people with BPD dysfunctional mentalization is more apparent in the emergence of unusual alternative strategies (hyper-mentalizing) than in the loss of the capacity per se (no mentalizing or under-mentalizing). This is hardly surprising, since individuals with BPD present quite differently from people with ASDs, where under-mentalization is most commonly observed. As opposed to individuals with schizophrenia (discussed earlier), it is unlikely that hyper-mentalizing results from an inability to recognize mental states in self and others (under-mentalizing). Most studies support the notion that those with BPD are able to recognize mental states in self and others, with some studies (Fertuck *et al.*, 2009) even demonstrating enhanced capacity to identify the mental state of others from expressions in the eye region of the face among BPD individuals. Thus, hyper-mentalization in people with BPD is not the result of mindblindness; rather, individuals with BPD tend to struggle with the integration and differentiation of mental states, especially under conditions of high emotional arousal. Therefore, mentalizing deficits in BPD seem to operate at a higher metacognitive level than at a lower perceptual level (Semerari *et al.*, 2005).

The tendency for borderline adolescents to hyper-mentalize may be attributable to the trauma histories associated with BPD (Zanarini, 2000; Zanarini *et al.*, 1989). Recent animal research suggests that early trauma may permanently affect the hypothalamic-pituitary-adrenal (HPA) axis (Oitzl *et al.*, 2000). Research with traumatized children and adult female victims of childhood sexual abuse has also demonstrated persistent changes in the HPA axis (Heim *et al.*, 2000, 2001). Indeed, abnormal stress responsiveness (Rinne *et al.*, 2002) has been demonstrated in adults with BPD. Increased stress responsiveness in turn affects mentalizing capacity. A recent study (Smeets *et al.*, 2009) used the MASC to show that high cortisol responding women make more mentalizing errors – in particular due to a tendency to hyper-mentalize – after stress induction, thereby demonstrating that stress responsiveness modulates mentalizing.

It is also possible that hyper-mentalization may develop not only in the presence of abuse, but in the absence of the protective factors that dampen the affects of stress – most notably secure attachment (see Chapter 1 this volume by Fonagy & Allison). In the developmental model of mentalization, attachment security provides the infant with the context to develop her own mentalizing capacity through the caregiver's capacity to treat her as a psychological agent (see Sharp & Fonagy, 2008a for a discussion). It is possible to draw parallels between this developmental model of BPD and Linehan's (1993) notion that an invalidating environment precedes BPD.

While exposure to chronic and episodic life stress and an invalidating, insecure attachment context are environmental contributors to the development of hyper-mentalizing, it is certainly possible that interpersonal hyper-sensitivity is inherited. Gunderson (2007) noted that the interpersonal style of BPD has a familial incidence similar to the affective instability and impulsivity phenotypes of BPD. The fact that mentalizing has known neural correlates (Frith & Frith, 1999; Frith & Wolpert, 2004) supports the notion of hyper-mentalizing as a neurocognitive endophenotype relating a genetic predisposition to the behavioural phenotype of disturbed interpersonal relationships. While pharmacological treatment is effective in reducing symptoms of impulsivity and affective instability in people with BPD, no 'relationship medication' has been discovered. This reality emphasizes the importance of treatment approaches described in this book for beginning to ameliorate the genetic and/or environmentally determined relational endophenotype described here.

A theory of nasty minds

Distorted mentalizing in externalizing behaviour problems

Externalizing behaviour problems refer to a broad range of disruptive antisocial behaviours captured by the diagnoses of conduct disorder and oppositional defiant disorder (American Psychiatric Association, 2000). The prevalence rates of externalizing disorders (including disorders such as conduct disorder and oppositional defiant disorder) are currently estimated to be 10 per cent (and rising) in the US (Tcheremissine *et al.*, 2004), with a recent epidemiological study suggesting a lifetime prevalence of 19.6 per cent for externalizing behaviour problems in youth (vs. 14.3 per cent for depression; Merikangas *et al.*, 2010). In a community sample of British children, the British Child and Adolescent Mental Health Survey in 1999 estimated the prevalence of *DSM-IV* disruptive disorder slightly lower, at 5.9 per cent (American Psychiatric Association, 2000; Ford *et al.*, 2003).

One of the hallmark features of externalizing problems is interpersonal difficulties. Children with externalizing problems tend to have poor relationships with peers (Vitaro *et al.*, 2001) and parents (Greenberg *et al.*, 1991). Therefore, social-cognitive theories provide a useful framework for understanding and addressing interpersonal difficulties in these children. One of the main social-cognitive approaches has been that of Dodge and colleagues (Dodge *et al.*, 2002; Mize & Pettit, 2008). This research has shown that children with conduct problems tend to have deficits in all aspects of social information processing, including: the encoding of social information; interpretation/representation about the causes of events; clarification of desired outcomes of interactions; response decision and behavioural enactment. Of particular interest from a mentalizing perspective is the tendency of children with conduct problems to attribute hostile intentions to others in ambiguous situations. Presumably then, these children respond aggressively to others because they expect aggression from others, even in the absence of evidence.

Other approaches to studying the relation between mentalization and externalizing problems have employed ToM (Happé & Frith, 1996; Hughes *et al.*, 1998; Sharp, 2008; Sutton *et al.*, 2000) and distorted mentalizing (Sharp *et al.*, 2006, 2007). While mentalizing deficits could not be demonstrated through false-belief tasks in preschool children (Happé & Frith,

1996; Hughes *et al.*, 1998), we demonstrated distorted mentalizing in this group of children in the 7 to 11 year age range (Sharp *et al.*, 2006, 2007). More specifically, children with conduct problems showed an overly positive mentalizing style in interpreting others' thoughts in relation to themselves. This style of mentalizing was found to be more apparent in children of mothers who engaged in reduced mentalizing, and furthermore predicts the onset of conduct problems over time (Ha *et al.*, 2011).

In another study (Sharp, 2008), we demonstrated deficits in emotion understanding in 7 to 11 year olds with externalizing problems using a task requiring children to read the emotions in the eye region of the face (Child's Eye Task; Baron-Cohen *et al.*, 2001). Using the adult version of this test, Richell *et al.* (2003) failed to demonstrate similar deficits in emotion understanding in adult psychopaths, suggesting that cortical regions may compensate during development for the early reduced (but not absent) amygdala functioning which usually accompanies emotion understanding. In other words, it is possible that those with externalizing behaviour problems learn to compensate for deficits in emotion understanding over time, but that this capacity for giving socially desirable responses is not yet developed in pre-adolescent children with externalizing problems.

While the above studies are informative in increasing our understanding of mentalizing deficits associated with externalizing problems, they are limited in that they make use of experimental tasks that assess 'off-line' mentalizing. That is, tasks that typically require responses to hypothetical scenarios and are not administered in real time. They do not sample actual social interactions and are therefore unlikely to elicit full emotional and behavioural engagement. In a recent study (Sharp *et al.*, 2011), we addressed this limitation by having boys with and without externalizing problems play a trust game in real time. One player (the Investor) was endowed with a certain amount of money. The Investor could keep all of the money or decide to 'invest' some amount with a partner (the Trustee). The amount invested was tripled as it was sent to the Trustee, who then decided what portion to return to the Investor. Two behavioural variables were of interest in this task. By investing in a partner, the Investor displayed 'trust' (making himself vulnerable by taking action that creates incentives for the other party to exploit him), while the Trustee displays 'trustworthiness' (reciprocity). It is assumed that trust and trustworthiness require the capacity to detect or predict the intentions of the other player (Falk & Fischbacher, 2006). Trust behaviour also requires the capacity to view the game from the other player's perspective (Singer & Fehr, 2005). Mentalizing, which is human intentionality exercised in social settings, therefore lies at the basis of trust behaviour. Given known mentalizing problems associated with externalizing problems (discussed earlier), it was not surprising that boys with externalizing problems showed anomalies in trust behaviour, especially with regard to trustworthiness. Moreover, trust and trustworthiness were related to social-cognitive reasoning during behavioural decision making, such that Investors who reported malevolent intentions were more likely to be in the externalizing group. These boys were also more likely to view the return offers from Trustees as unfair, indicating that they read malevolence in the intentions of others. Interestingly, in this group of adolescent boys, trust and trustworthiness did not relate to mentalizing capacity as measured by the Child's Eye Task, a more 'off-line' mentalizing task. This is interesting because it suggests that some components of mentalizing can only be accessed or measured during real-time, real-life interaction as in a social exchange game. The study is additionally informative in that it empirically complements early theoretical work on the importance of trust (Erikson, 1950) and, therefore, attachment (Bowlby, 1973, 1980) in the development of optimal interpersonal functioning.

Pseudo-mentalizing: if it looks like a duck . . .

While the tendency to attribute malevolent intentions to self and others as discussed above may characterize the interpersonal interactions of children with externalizing behaviour problems, Sutton *et al.* (2000) demonstrated mentalizing problems of another kind in the most severe subgroup of children with externalizing problems. They set out to explore mentalizing problems in externalizing disorder by using tests of ToM appropriate for middle school age children and showed no relation between mentalizing and externalizing behaviour problems. In fact, they showed that bullies, who typically engage in more severe indirect and proactive aggression, are actually advanced in their mentalizing skills. They suggested that these children become skilled mindreaders in response to aversive environments characterized by harsh and inconsistent discipline. This tendency to engage in mindreading, that looks like mentalizing but lacks some of the essential features of genuine mentalizing, is referred to as pseudo-mentalizing (Allen *et al.*, 2008). As such, pseudo-mentalizing involves the use of mentalizing to manipulate or control behaviour, as opposed to genuine mentalizing, which reflects true curiosity and a general respect for the minds of others.

Another example of pseudo-mentalizing in childhood disorder can be found in the work of Crick and Grotpeter (1996). These authors showed that relationally aggressive girls tend to victimize their friends by eliciting intimacy and encouraging disclosure in order to acquire control, which is then used to manipulate the relationship by threatening to expose their friends' secrets. A certain level of mentalizing skill is required for such sophisticated social manipulation. However, we refrain from calling this mentalizing, since mentalizing in the above case is used for goals that do not enhance the capacity for optimal interpersonal functioning.

Perhaps one of the best examples of pseudo-mentalizing is the case of psychopathy. As mentioned before, there is some evidence that adolescent and adult psychopaths can mindread, but that this mindreading is accounted for by the 'thinking' (prefrontal) regions of the brain rather than the 'feeling' (amygdala) regions of the brain (Richell *et al.*, 2003; Sharp, 2008). Blair and co-workers (2006) provide a helpful framework for understanding the ability of psychopaths to fake understanding mental states in others. Blair and colleagues distinguish between perspective taking and empathy. They define empathy as an affective response more appropriate to someone else's situation than one's own. Because empathy entails an emotional response to someone else's state, it can be seen as a consequence of roletaking. Roletaking, in turn, requires the representation of another's internal state and thus involves mentalizing. As such, empathy is an emotional response to a representation of another's internal state. While psychopaths may have no trouble in the latter, evidence suggests that they have difficulties with empathizing. For instance, it was shown that young adolescents with psychopathic tendencies report reduced responsiveness to sad and fearful but not angry facial expressions (Blair & Coles, 2001; Stevens *et al.*, 2001) and show less responsiveness to these stimuli as measured by electrodermal responses (Blair, 1999). Blair's work attests to a selective impairment in the mentalizing of sad and fearful stimuli related to reduced amygdala functioning. The amydala is critical for stimulus reinforcement learning and feeding reinforcement expectance information forward to the orbital frontal cortex allowing good decision making to occur (Blair, 2010). Both of these processes are disrupted in youth with psychopathic traits, which prohibits socializing through reinforcement from parents, peers or other adults. As Cleckley (1941) originally noted in his landmark book, psychopaths wear a 'mask of sanity': they appear to mentalize, but, without the associated amygdala responses, in truth, they are pseudo-mentalizing.

Mentalizing and internalizing problems

A view from social information processing theory

Anxiety disorders have recently been placed within the framework of social cognition by Banerjee (2008), who combines Beck and Clark's (1997) cognitive model of anxiety with Daleiden and Vasey's (1997) social information processing model. In particular, he suggests that social cognition in children with anxiety disorders is characterized by hypervigilance with regard to possible threat and negative evaluations of social events and past encounters, and that this hypervigilance is a consequence of ToM deficits. In this regard, Frith *et al.* (1994) found that children with social anxiety experienced social skills deficits in tasks that required mentalizing. Similarly, Banerjee and Watling (2004, 2010) found that socially anxious children, while likely to engage in self-presentation strategies like non-anxious children, failed to modify those strategies with regard to their audience, implying difficulty in the detection of their social partners' preferences. These studies indicate that anxious youth experience 'difficulty with understanding and effectively managing social situations involving multiple mental states' (Banerjee, 2008: 253). This mentalizing or ToM deficit has two outcomes. First, it leads to the social skills deficits observed in these children. Second, it underlies the hypervigilance these children display in the absence of knowledge about the minds of others. In suggesting that this basic ToM deficit may underlie later social information processing biases (threat perception), Banerjee's model is intriguing, because it links deficit approaches in social cognition to distortion approaches in the same way earlier described for schizophrenia.

Approaches to understanding the social deficits associated with depression in children and adolescents have, like anxiety disorder research, relied mostly on the use of social information processing frameworks. To our knowledge, no studies have directly explored the relation between depression and ToM in children and adolescents. Similarly, information about ToM in depressed adults is extremely limited and, as such, inconclusive. One study by Kettle *et al.* (2008) concluded that adults diagnosed with depression do not differ from normal controls with regard to ToM ability while Lee *et al.* (2005) concluded that adult women with depression performed more poorly on a measure of ToM (Eyes Task) compared to normal controls.

Despite the paucity and disagreement of existing studies directly exploring ToM and depression, some hypotheses about their relation can be informed by work relating to other constructs including mindfulness and social information processing. Allen (2003), for instance, suggests that mindfulness based treatment is basically the 'clinical application of mentalizing' (p. 104) and, thus, the utility of mindfulness for treating depression implies that depression is related to some deficit in mentalization. Similarly, a literature review conducted by Kyte and Goodyer (2008) highlights studies that, though not directly assessing mentalization or ToM, place childhood and adolescent depression within a social cognitive framework. Specifically, they present literature linking depression to impairment in multiple domains affecting social information processing including: negative self-schemas (Zupan *et al.*, 1987); selectively focused attention and recall on negative stimuli (Hammen & Zupan, 1984); maladaptive and negative attributional style (Muris *et al.*, 2001; Voelz *et al.*, 2003); rumination (Nolen-Hoeksema, 2000; Park *et al.*, 2004); and impulsive and suboptimal decision making (Kyte *et al.*, 2005). An integration of this literature with the more traditional theory of mind or mentalizing literature would considerably move forward the study of social-cognitive deficits associated with depression. As of yet, this integration has not taken place.

Conclusion

The goal of this chapter was to review mentalizing problems in children and adolescents using a taxonomy of mentalizing which includes several types of mentalizing difficulties: no mentalizing, under-mentalizing, hyper-mentalizing, pseudo-mentalizing and distorted mentalizing. In short, we reviewed literature demonstrating no or under-mentalizing in children with ASDs. We discussed how similar mentalizing failures were apparent in adolescents or young adults with schizophrenia, but that such under-mentalizing preceded a process by which intentions were attributed to others inappropriately (hyper-mentalizing). We discussed a new study demonstrating hyper-mentalizing (in the absence of under-mentalizing) in adolescents with BPD. We also illustrated that depending on the mentalizing task, either distorted or under-mentalizing could be demonstrated in pre-adolescent children with conduct problems, while pseudo-mentalizing appears to be present in the most conduct disturbed group of children, namely those with psychopathic traits.

Together, the research discussed in this chapter clearly establishes mentalizing as an important endophenotype to be targeted in treatment, thereby providing a clear rationale for the treatment approaches described in this book. Second, it illuminates how different aspects of mentalizing are reflected in the heterogeneity of different childhood disorders. Mentalizing is not all of one piece, but represents an uneven distribution of capacities depending on three factors: the developmental phase of the child; the characteristics of the disorder; and the particular mentalizing capacity being studied. Perhaps then, the development of mentalizing and its uneven distribution within and across disorders is well described by the Piagetian concept of 'horizontal decolage'. Piaget (1952) used the term to describe inconsistent performance in problems requiring the same cognitive processes. In the same way, in mental health problems in children and adolescents we see inconsistent mentalizing performance across different tasks for what we assume to be an underlying, general deficit in mentalizing capacity.

References

Aldred, C., Green, J., & Adams, C. (2004). A new social communication intervention for children with autism: Pilot randomised controlled treatment study suggesting effectiveness. *Journal of Child Psychology and Psychiatry*, 45(8), 1420–1430.

Allen, J. (2002). *Traumatic attachments*. New York: Wiley.

Allen, J. G. (2003). Mentalizing. *Bulletin of the Menninger Clinic*, 67(2), 91–112.

Allen, J. (2006). Mentalizing in practice. In J. Allen & P. Fonagy (Eds.), *Handbook of mentalization-based treatment* (pp. 1–24). Chichester: Wiley.

Allen, J., Fonagy, P., & Bateman, A. W. (2008). *Mentalizing in clinical practice*. Washington: American Psychiatric Publishing.

American Psychiatric Association (2000). *Diagnostic and statistical manual of mental disorders* (4th ed., text revision). Washington, DC: American Psychiatric Association.

Banerjee, R. (2008). Social cognition and anxiety in children. In C. Sharp, P. Fonagy & I. Goodyer (Eds.), *Social cognition and developmental psychopathology* (pp. 239–269). New York: Oxford University Press.

Banerjee, R., & Watling, D. (2004). Social anxiety and depressive symptoms in childhood: Models of distinctive pathways. Presented at the British Psychological Association Annual Conference, Imperial College, University of London.

Banerjee, R., & Watling, D. (2010). Self-presentational features in childhood social anxiety. *Journal of Anxiety Disorders*, 24(1), 34–41.

Baron-Cohen, S. (1987). Autism and symbolic play. *British Journal of Developmental Psychology*, 5(2), 139–148.

Baron-Cohen, S. (1989). Are autistic children 'behaviorists'? An examination of their mental-physical and appearance-reality distinctions. *Journal of Autism and Developmental Disorders*, 19(4), 579–600.

Baron-Cohen, S. (1991). Do people with autism understand what causes emotion? *Child Development*, 62, 385–395.

Baron-Cohen, S. (1995). *Mindblindness: An essay on autism and theory of mind.* Cambridge, MA: MIT Press.

Baron-Cohen, S., & Goodhart, F. (1994). The 'seeing leads to knowing' deficit in autism: The Pratt and Bryant probe. *British Journal of Developmental Psychology*, 12, 397–402.

Baron-Cohen, S., & Wheelright, S. (2004). The empathy quotient: An investigation of adults with Asperger syndrome or high functioning autism, and normal sex differences. *Journal of Autism and Developmental Disorders*, 34(2), 163–175.

Baron-Cohen, S., Leslie, A. M., & Frith, U. (1985). Does the autistic child have a 'theory of mind'? *Cognition*, 21(1), 37–46.

Baron-Cohen, S., Ring, H., Moriarty, J., Schmitz, B., Costa, D., & Ell, P. (1994). Recognition of mental state terms. Clinical findings in children with autism and a functional neuroimaging study of normal adults. *British Journal of Psychiatry*, 165(5), 640–649.

Baron-Cohen, S., Wheelwright, S., Hill, J., Raste, Y., & Plumb, I. (2001). The 'Reading the mind in the eyes' Test revised version: A study with normal adults, and adults with Asperger syndrome or high-functioning autism. *Journal of Child Psychology and Psychiatry and Allied Disciplines*, 42(2), 241–251.

Baron-Cohen, S., Richler, J., Bisarya, D., Gurunathan, N., & Wheelright, S. (2003). The systemizing quotient: An investigation of adults with Asperger syndrome or high-functioning autism, and normal sex differences. *Philosophical Transactions of the Royal Society*, Series B, special issue on 'Autism: Mind and brain' 358, 361–374.

Bateman, A., & Fonagy, P. (2004). *Psychotherapy for borderline personality disorder: Mentalization-based treatment*. Oxford: Oxford University Press.

Beck, A. T., & Clark, D. A. (1997). An information processing model of anxiety: Automatic and strategic processes. *Behaviour Research and Therapy*, 35(1), 49–58.

Belmonte, M. K. (2008). Does the experimental scientist have a 'theory of mind'? *Review of General Psychology*, 12(2), 192–204.

Blair, R. J. R. (1999). Responsiveness to distress cues in the child with psychopathic tendencies. *Personality and Individual Differences*, 27(1), 135–145.

Blair, R. J. (2010). Neuroimaging of psychopathy and antisocial behavior: A targeted review. *Current Psychiatry Reports*, 12(1), 76–82.

Blair, R. J. R., & Coles, M. (2001). Expression recognition and behavioural problems in early adolescence. *Cognitive Development*, 15(4), 421–434.

Blair, R. J., Peschardt, K. S., Budhani, S., Mitchell, D. G., & Pine, D. S. (2006). The development of psychopathy. *Journal of Child Psychology and Psychiatry*, 47(3/4), 262–275.

Bowlby, J. (1973). *Attachment and loss, Vol. 2: Separation: Anxiety and anger*. New York: Basic Books.

Bowlby, J. (1980). *Attachment and loss, Vol. 3: Loss, sadness and depression*. London: Hogarth Press.

Charman, T., & Baron-Cohen, S. (1997). Brief report: Prompted pretend play in autism. *Journal of Autism and Developmental Disorders*, 27(3), 325–332.

Charman, T., Swettenham, J., Baron-Cohen, S., Cox, A., Baird, G., & Drew, A. (1997). Infants with autism: An investigation of empathy, pretend play, joint attention, and imitation. *Developmental Psychology*, 33(5), 781–789.

Chomsky, N. (1980). *Rules and representations*. New York: Columbia University Press.

Cleckley, H. (1941). *The mask of sanity*. St. Louis, MO: Mosby.

Crick, N. R., & Grotpeter, J. K. (1996). Relational aggression, gender, and social-psychological adjustment. *Child Development*, 66, 710–722.

Daleiden, E. L., & Vasey, M. W. (1997). An information-processing perspective on childhood anxiety. *Clinical Psychology Review*, 17(4), 407–429.

Dodge, K. A., Laird, R., Lochman, J. E., Zelli, A., & Conduct Problems Prevention Research Group, U. S. (2002). Multidimensional latent-construct analysis of children's social information processing patterns: Correlations with aggressive behavior problems. *Psychological Assessment*, 14(1), 60–73.

Dziobek, I., Fleck, S., Kalbe, E., Rogers, K., Hassenstab, J., Brand, M., *et al.* (2006). Introducing MASC: A movie for the assessment of social cognition. *Journal of Autism and Developmental Disorders*, 36(5), 623–636.

Erikson, E. (1950). *Childhood in society*. New York: Norton.

Falk, A., & Fischbacher, U. (2006). A theory of reciprocity. *Games and Economic Behavior*, 54(2), 293–315.

Fertuck, E. A., Jekal, A., Song, I., Wyman, B., Morris, M. C., Wilson, S., *et al.* (2009). Enhanced 'Reading the Mind in the Eyes' in borderline personality disorder compared to healthy controls. *Psychological Medicine*, 39(12), 1979–1988.

Ford, T., Goodman, R., & Meltzer, H. (2003). The British Child and Adolescent Mental Health Survey 1999: The prevalence of DSM-IV disorders. *Journal of the American Academy of Child & Adolescent Psychiatry*, 42(10), 1203–1211.

Frith, C. D., & Frith, U. (1999). Interacting minds – a biological basis. *Science*, 286(5445), 1692–1695.

Frith, C. D., & Wolpert, D. M. (2004). *The neuroscience of social interaction:*

Decoding, imitating and influencing the actions of others. Oxford: Oxford University Press.

Frith, U., & Happé, F. (1994). Autism: Beyond 'theory of mind'. *Cognition*, 50(1–3), 115–132.

Frith, U., Happé, F., & Siddons, F. (1994). Autism and theory of mind in everyday life. *Social Development*, 3(2), 108–124.

Greenberg, M. T., Speltz, M. L., DeKlyen, M., & Endriga, M.C. (1991). Attachment security in pre-schoolers with and without externalizing behaviour problems: A replication. *Development and Psychopathology*, 3, 413–430.

Gunderson, J. G. (2007). Disturbed relationships as a phenotype for borderline personality disorder. *American Journal of Psychiatry*, 164(11), 1637–1640.

Ha, C., Sharp, C., & Goodyer, I.M. (2011). The role of child and parental mentalizing for the development of conduct problems over time. *European Journal of Child and Adolescent Psychiatry*, 20, 291–300.

Hammen, C., & Zupan, B. A. (1984). Self-schemas, depression, and the processing of personal information in children. *Journal of Experimental Child Psychology*, 37(3), 598–608.

Happé, F. G. E., & Frith, U. (1996). Theory of mind and social impairment in children with conduct disorder. *British Journal of Developmental Psychology*, 14(4), 385–398.

Harrington, L., Langdon, R., Siegert, R. J., & McClure, J. (2005). Schizophrenia, theory of mind, and persecutory delusions. *Cognitive Neuropsychiatry*, 10(2), 87–104.

Heim, C., Newport, D. J., Heit, S., Graham, Y. P., Wilcox, M., Bonsall, R., *et al.* (2000). Pituitary-adrenal and autonomic respones to stress in women after sexual and physical abuse in childhood. *JAMA*, 284, 592–597.

Heim, C., Newport, D. J., Bonsall, R., Miller, A. H., & Nemeroff, C. B. (2001). Altered pituitary-adrenal axis responses to provocative challenge tests in adult survivors of childhood abuse. *American Journal of Psychiatry*, 158, 575–581.

Hobson, R. P., & Lee, A. (1999). Imitation and identification in autism. *Journal of Child Psychology and Psychiatry*, 40(4), 649–659.

Howlin, P., Gordon, R. K., Pasco, G., Wade, A., & Charman, T. (2007). The effectiveness of Picture Exchange Communication System (PECS) training for teachers of children with autism: A pragmatic, group randomised controlled trial. *Journal of Child Psychology and Psychiatry*, 48(5), 473–481.

Hughes, C., Dunn, J., & White, A. (1998). Trick or treat? Uneven understanding of mind and emotion and executive dysfunction in 'hard-to-manage' preschoolers. *Journal of Child Psychology and Psychiatry and Allied Disciplines*, 39(7), 981–994.

Kasari, C., Freeman, S., & Paparella, T. (2006). Joint attention and symbolic play in young children with autism: A randomized controlled intervention study. *Journal of Child Psychology and Psychiatry*, 47(6), 611–620.

Kettle, J. L., O'Brien-Simpson, L., & Allen, N. B. (2008). Impaired theory of mind in first-episode schizophrenia: Comparison with community, university and depressed controls. *Schizophrenia Research*, 99(1–3), 96–102.

Kington, J. M., Jones, L. A., Watt, A. A., Hopkin, E. J., & Williams, J. J. (2000). Impaired eye expression recognition in schizophrenia. *Journal of Psychiatric Research*, 34(4–5), 341–347.

Krohn, A. J. (1974). Borderline 'empathy' and differentiation of object representations: A contribution to the psychology of object relations. *International Journal of Psychiatry*, 3, 142–165.

Kyte, Z., & Goodyer, I. (2008). Social cognition in depressed children and adolescents. In C. Sharp, P. Fonagy, I. Goodyer, C. Sharp, P. Fonagy & I. Goodyer (Eds.), *Social cognition and developmental psychopathology* (pp. 201–237). New York: Oxford University Press.

Kyte, Z. A., Goodyer, I. M., & Sahakian, B. J. (2005). Selected executive skills in adolescents with recent first episode major depression. *Journal of Child Psychology and Psychiatry*, 46(9), 995–1005.

Langdon, R. (2003). Theory of mind and social dysfunction: Psychotic solipsism versus autistic asociality. In B. Repacholi & V. Slaughter (Eds.), *Individual differences in theory of mind: Implications for typical and atypical development* (pp. 241–269). New York: Psychology Press.

Langdon, R. (2005). Theory of mind in schizophrenia. In B. F. Malle & S. D. Hodges (Eds.), *Other minds: How humans bridge the divide between self and others* (pp. 333–342). New York: Guilford Press.

Langdon, R., & Brock, J. (2008). Hypo- or hyper-mentalizing: It all depends upon what one means by 'mentalizing'. *Behavioral and Brain Sciences*, 31(3), 274–275.

Langdon, R., & Coltheart, M. (2001). Visual perspective-taking and schizotypy: Evidence for a simulation-based account of mentalizing in normal adults. *Cognition*, 82(1), 1–26.

Langdon, R., Coltheart, M., Ward, P. B., & Catts, S. V. (2001). Visual and cognitive perspective-taking impairments in schizophrenia: A failure of allocentric simulation? *Cognitive Neuropsychiatry*, 6(4), 241–269.

Langdon, R., Coltheart, M., & Ward, P. B. (2006). Empathetic perspective-taking is impaired in schizophrenia: Evidence from a study of emotion attribution and theory of mind. *Cognitive Neuropsychiatry*, 11(2), 133–155.

Lee, L., Harkness, K., Sabbagh, M., & Jacobson, J. (2005). Mental state decoding abilities in clinical depression. *Journal of Affective Disorders*, 86(2–3), 247–258.

Leekam, S. R., & Perner, J. (1991). Does the autistic child have a metarepresentational deficit? *Cognition*, 40(3), 203–218.

Leudar, I., & Costall, A. (2010). *Against theory of mind.* Basingstoke: Macmillan.

Linehan, M. M. (1993). *Cognitive-behavioral treatment of borderline personality disorder*. New York: Guilford Press.

Loveland, K., & Tunali, B. (1994). Narrative language in autism and the theory of affect in autism. *Development and Psychopathology*, 6, 433–444.

Merikangas, K.R., He, J., Burstein, M., Swanson, S., Avenevoli, S., Cui, L., *et al.* (2010). Lifetime prevalence of mental disorders in U.S. adolescents: Results from the National Comorbidity Survey Replication-Adolescent Supplement (NCS-A). *Journal of the American Academy of Child and Adolescent Psychiatry*, 49(10), 980–989.

Mize, J., & Pettit, G. S. (2008). Social information processing and the development of conduct problems in children and adoelscents: Looking beneath the surface. In C. Sharp, P. Fonagy & I. M. Goodyer (Eds.), *Social cognition and developmental psychopathology* (pp. 141–174). Oxford: Oxford University Press.

Montag, C., Ehrlich, A., Neuhaus, K., Dziobek, I., Heekeren, H. R., Heinz, A., *et al.* (2009). Theory of mind impairments in euthymic bipolar patients. *Journal of Affective Disorders*, 123(1–3), 264–269.

Muris, P., Schmidt, H., Lambrichs, R., & Meesters, C. (2001). Protective and vulnerability factors of depression in normal adolescents. *Behaviour Research and Therapy*, 39(5), 555–565.

Nesse, R. M. (2004). Cliff-edged fitness functions and the persistence of schizophrenia. *Behavioural and Brain Sciences*, 27, 862–863.

Nolen-Hoeksema, S. (2000). The role of rumination in depressive disorders and mixed anxiety/depressive symptoms. *Journal of Abnormal Psychology*, 109(3), 504–511.

Oitzl, M. S., Workel, J. O., Fluttert, M., Frosch, F., & De Kloet, E. R. (2000). Maternal deprivation affects behaviour from youth to senescence: Amplication of individual differences in spatial learning and memory in senescence Brown Norway rats. *European Journal of Neuroscience*, 12, 3771–3780.

Park, R. J., Goodyer, I. M., & Teasdale, J. D. (2004). Effects of induced rumination and distraction on mood and overgeneral autobiographical memory in adolescent major depressive disorder and controls. *Journal of Child Psychology and Psychiatry*, 45(5), 996–1006.

Piaget, J. (1952). *The child's conception of number*. New York: Humanities Press.

Richell, R. A., Mitchell, D. G., Newman, C., Leonard, A., Baron-Cohen, S., & Blair, R. J. (2003). Theory of mind and psychopathy: Can psychopathic individuals read the 'language of the eyes'? *Neuropsychologia*, 41(5), 523–526.

Rinne, T., de Kloet, E. R., Wouters, L., Goekoop, J. G., DeRijk, R. H., & van den Brink, W. (2002). Hyperresponsiveness of hypothalamic-pituitary-adrenal axis to combined dexamethasone/corticotropin-releasing hormone challenge in female borderline personality disorder subjects with a history of sustained childhood abuse. *Biological Psychiatry*, 52(11), 1102–1112.

Roeyers, H., Van Oost, P., & Bothuyne, S. (1998). Immediate imitation and joint attention in young children with autism. *Developmental Psychopathology*, 10(3), 441–450.

Russell, J., & Jarrold, C. (1999). Memory for actions in children with autism: Self versus other. *Cognitive Neuropsychiatry*, 4(4), 303–331.

Semerari, A., Carcione, A., Dimaggio, G., Nicolo, G., Pedone, R., & Procacci, M. (2005). Metarepresentative functions in borderline personality disorder. *Journal of Personality Disorders*, 19(6), 690–710.

Sharp, C. (2006). Mentalizing problems in childhood disorders. In J. G. Allen & P. Fonagy (Eds.), *Handbook of mentalization-based treatments* (pp. 101–121). Chichester: Wiley.

Sharp, C. (2008). Theory of mind and conduct problems in children: Deficits in reading the 'emotions of the eyes'. *Cognition and Emotion*, 22(6), 1149–1158.

Sharp, C., & Fonagy, P. (2008a). The parent's capacity to treat the child as a psychological agent: Constructs, measures and implications for developmental psychopathology. *Social Development*, 17(3), 737–754.

Sharp, C., & Fonagy, P. (2008b). Social cognition and attachment-related disorders. In C. Sharp, P. Fonagy & I. Goodyer (Eds.), *Social cognition and developmental psychopathology* (pp. 269–302). Oxford: Oxford University Press.

Sharp, C., Fonagy, P., & Goodyer, I. M. (2006). Imagining your child's mind: Psychosocial adjustment and mothers' ability to predict their children's attributional response styles. *British Journal of Developmental Psychology*, 24, 197–214.

Sharp, C., Croudace, T. J., & Goodyer, I. M. (2007). Biased mentalising in children aged 7–11: Latent class confirmation of response styles to social scenarios and associations with psychopathology. *Social Development*, 16(1), 81–202.

Sharp, C., Ha, C., & Fonagy, P. (2011). Get them before they get you: Trust, trustworthiness and social cognition in boys with and without externalizing behavior problems. *Development and Psychopathology*, 23, 647–658.

Sharp, C., Pane, H., Ha, C., Venta, A., Patel, A., Sturek, J., *et al.* (2011). Theory of mind and emotion regulation difficulties in adolescents with borderline traits. *Journal of the American Academy of Child and Adolescent Psychiatry*, 50, 563–573.

Singer, T., & Fehr, E. (2005). The neuroeconomics of mindreading and emphathy. *AEA Papers and Proceedings*, 95(2), 340–345.

Smeets, T., Dziobek, I., & Wolf, O. T. (2009). Social cognition under stress: Differential effects of stress-induced cortisol elevations in healthy young men and women. *Hormones and Behavior*, 55(4), 507–513.

Smith, I. M., & Bryson, S. E. (1994). Imitation and action in autism: A critical review. *Psychological Bulletin*, 116(2), 259–273.

Stevens, D., Charman, T., & Blair, R. J. R. (2001). Recognition of emotion in facial expressions and vocal tones in children with psychopathic tendencies. *Journal of Genetic Psychology*, 162(2), 201–211.

Sutton, J., Reeves, M., & Keogh, E. (2000). Disruptive behaviour, avoidance of responsibility and theory of mind. *British Journal of Developmental Psychology*, 18(Pt 1), 1–11.

Tcheremissine, O. V., Cherek, D. R., & Lane, S. D. (2004). Psychopharmacology of conduct disorder: current progress and future directions. *Expert Opinion on Pharmacotherapy*, 5(5), 1109–1116.

Tordjman, S. (2008). Reunifying autism and early-onset schizophrenia in terms of social communication disorders. *Behavioral and Brain Sciences*, 31(3), 278–279.

Vitaro, F., Tremblay, R.E., & Bykowski, W.M. (2001). Friends, friendships and conduct disorders. In J. Hill & B. Maughan (Eds.), *Conduct disorders in childhood and adolescence* (pp. 346–376). Cambridge: Cambridge University Press.

Voelz, Z. R., Haeffel, G. J., Joiner, T. R., & Wagner, K. (2003). Reducing hope-essness: The interaction [sic] of enhancing and depressogenic attributional styles for positive and negative life events among youth psychiatric inpatients. *Behaviour Research and Therapy*, 41(10), 1183–1198.

Volkmar, F., Chawarska, K., & Klin, A. (2005). Autism in infancy and early childhood. *Annual Review of Psychology*, 56, 315–336.

von Ceumern-Lindenstjerna, I. A., Brunner, R., Parzer, P., Mundt, C., Fiedler, P., & Resch, F. (2010). Initial orienting to emotional faces in female adolescents with borderline personality disorder. *Psychopathology*, 43(2), 79–87.

Wimmer, H., Hogrefe, G. J., & Perner, J. (1988). Children's understanding of informational access as a source of knowledge. *Child Development*, 59, 386–396.

Yirmiya, N., & Shulman, C. (1996). Seriation, conservation, and theory of mind abilities in individuals with autism, individuals with mental retardation, and normally developing children. *Child Development*, 67(5), 2045–2059.

Zanarini, M. C. (2000). Childhood experiences associated with the development of borderline personality disorder. *Psychiatric Clinics of North America*, 23(1), 89–101.

Zanarini, M. C., Gunderson, J. G., Marino, M. F., Schwartz, E. O., & Frankenburg, F. R. (1989). Childhood experiences of borderline patients. *Comprehensive Psychiatry*, 30(1), 18–25.

Zupan, B. A., Hammen, C., & Jaenicke, C. (1987). The effects of current mood and prior depressive history on self-schematic processing in children. *Journal of Experimental Child Psychology*, 43(1), 149–158.

Chapter 3

Measuring mentalization in children and young people

Ioanna Vrouva, Mary Target and Karin Ensink

Introduction

'How could anything be more familiar, and at the same time more weird, than a mind?' philosopher Dennett (1987) invites us to wonder. While physical objects can be directly perceived through their properties or attributes, psychological concepts such as emotions, cognitive capacities and personality traits are *private* and unobservable and therefore must be inferred and operationalized using sensitive methods. The measurement of mentalization is particularly challenging, as it involves making inferences not only about mental states that are largely unobservable, but also about one's ability to make inferences about various properties of this familiar, yet weird entity, the mind. It appears that measurement of mentalization typically requires a delicate synchronicity among three minds: that of the researcher, that of the participant, and that of a third, whom the participant is invited to understand.

As set out in Chapter 1, mentalization is considered a multidimensional concept, which can be thought to be organized along four polarities: self or other focused, automatic and implicit or controlled and explicit, cognitive or affective, and internal or external based (for a detailed description of each polarity, see Fonagy & Luyten, 2009). Furthermore, the capacity to mentalize may refer to various psychological processes such as desires, intentions, beliefs, needs, perceptions and attitudes, and is viewed as having both 'trait' and 'state' aspects. These are not consistent across domains and fluctuate in relation to emotional arousal and interpersonal experiences. It is also thought that mentalization is never fully acquired or maintained across all situations.

Despite the significant challenges inherent in the assessment of mentalization, it is important to develop valid and reliable measures so that we can: (a) assess the outcome of mentalization-based work and other therapies with children and adolescents; and (b) empirically test some theoretical propositions regarding the development of mentalization and its hypothesized role in mental health and psychopathology.

A note on definitional overlap

Mentalization is closely related to a family of adjacent constructs such as *reflective function (RF)*, *metacognition*, *theory of mind* (ToM), *mindreading*, *mindfulness*, *psychological mindedness*, *social or emotional understanding*, *socio-cognitive and socio-emotional abilities*, *social or emotional intelligence*, *affect consciousness*, *perspective taking* and *empathy* (Allen, 2003; Choi-Kain & Gunderson, 2008).

As mentalization overlaps theoretically with the above 'conceptual cousins', approaches to the measurement of these concepts can be relevant to the assessment of mentalization. Among these concepts, *reflective function* is particularly relevant. It can be thought of as demonstration of the capacity and propensity to consider both internal states (such as thoughts, feelings, beliefs and desires) and interpersonal processes in thinking about oneself and close relationships. In essence, reflective functioning is an operationalization for measuring the psychological function of mentalization, which organizes the experience of one's own and others' behaviour in terms of mental state constructs (Fonagy & Target, 2003).

Having broadly mapped the territory of the concept of mentalization, the aim of the remaining chapter is twofold. First, we briefly review existing approaches to the measurement of mentalization and its related constructs in children and adolescents. (The measurement of mentalizing in parents is beyond the scope of this chapter, but see Sharp & Fonagy, 2008 for a review of this work.) Second, we present three mentalization tasks developed at University College London (UCL) and – for the first two – the Anna Freud Centre, namely the Affect Task (AT; Fonagy *et al.*, 2000), the Reflective Functioning Scale for Children (CRFS; Ensink, 2003; Target *et al.*, 2001) and the Mentalizing Stories for Adolescents (MSA; Vrouva, 2010). We conclude by discussing both challenges and promising directions for future research.

Review of existing approaches to the measurement of mentalization and related concepts

From the first traces of intentionality to passing false belief tasks: measuring mentalization in young children

Without the medium of verbal communication as a basis for assessing the level of mentalization, research with infants has relied on observations of behaviour in natural or experimental conditions. There is a lot of evidence suggesting that infants are implicitly aware of others' mental states, for instance they are capable of tracking another's attention (Gergely *et al.*, 1995; see also Chapter 1 of this volume).

For preschool age children, standard theory of mind (ToM) tasks were developed to assess children's ability to take into account what others know and think. These tasks were primarily developed to investigate ToM deficits in autism. In parallel, investigators have also applied observational methods to collect data about young children's mentalizing abilities in naturalistic settings, focusing, for instance, on children's internal state talk or mental state language (Dunn *et al.*, 1991). This work was successfully pioneered by Judith Dunn and her colleagues at the Institute of Psychiatry in London and assessed mentalizing either during children's daily activities or in predetermined settings, taking into account topics such as children's pretend play, or use of humour. Dunn demonstrated that it is possible to systematize everyday family interaction for research purposes and showed that families differ remarkably in their use of mental state talk, and that for children these learning opportunities are vital for acquiring mentalization skills.

At the same time, affective understanding has become an important area of research. The choice of affective understanding measures for preschoolers is somewhat limited, but Denham's Affect Knowledge Test (AKT; Denham, 1986) is a puppet interview that has been widely used to assess socio-emotional understanding in this age group. The Berkeley puppet interview (BPI; Measelle *et al.*, 1998) was developed to assess young children's perceptions about themselves. A full review of the measures assessing these capacities in preschoolers is beyond the scope of this chapter, but interested readers are referred to the excellent review by Denham (2006).

Beyond false belief: measuring advanced ToM/mentalization in primary-school-aged children

While standard ToM tasks are mainly for preschool-age children, many of the non-standard and advanced measures are for a broader age range (Sprung, 2010). During the period of latency, significant changes in mentalization are expected as children acquire concrete and early formal operational thought structures (Steele & Steele, 2005). Between the ages of six and seven years, children develop second-order ToM abilities, namely they can understand that someone can hold a false belief about the belief of another character. Tasks assessing the ability to consider the intentions of the speaker in understanding everyday speech, in which what is said is not literally true, are known as third-order ToM tasks, due to their increased complexity.

Happé's Strange Stories (HSS; Happé, 1994), for instance, pitched at an eight-year-old level, assess explicit cognitive-linguistic aspects of ToM. The task involves interactions between two people, where one character says something which is not literally true, involving concepts such as a white lie, irony, persuasion, or misunderstanding. For example, a figure of speech story reads: 'Emma has a cough. All through lunch she coughs and coughs and coughs. Father says, "Poor Emma, you must have a frog in your throat!" Is it true, what Father says to Emma? Why does he say that?' To perform well at this task, children need to understand that communication depends on the intention of the speaker.

Tasks assessing explicit cognitive-linguistic aspects of ToM and in particular children's introspection skills, i.e. knowledge of their own thoughts, have been also developed (Sprung, 2010). For instance, Flavell *et al.* (2000) instructed their child participants to refrain from having any thoughts while sitting in a special 'no-thinking' chair. Afterwards, they asked several questions, including whether the children did or did not have any thoughts while sitting in the special no-thinking chair and whether it was hard or easy trying not to have any thoughts. This task samples mentalizing that is self-focused, cognitive, explicit but internal based, and taps a child's awareness of their own thought content.

Other ToM tasks assess the ability to process the appropriateness of behaviour in different social contexts. For instance, in the Faux Pas Test (Baron-Cohen *et al.*, 1999) children have to read short narratives of everyday interactions and answer questions specific to faux pas. One story reads: 'Sally has short blonde hair. She was at her Aunt Carol's house. The doorbell rang. It was Mary, a neighbour. Mary said "Hello," then looked at Sally and said, "Oh, I don't think I've met this little boy. What's your name?"' The children are asked whether anybody in the story said something that they should not have said.

Likewise, the Social Situations Task (Rogers *et al.*, 2006), assesses mental state attribution and social response prediction. This task presents children with short stories describing social situations incorporating behaviour that is either normative or peculiar (e.g. likely to shock/upset others), and children are required to classify the behaviour in each story as: (a) normal; (b) rather strange; (c) very strange; (d) shocking. As this task assesses children's ability to infer the impact of specific behaviours on the mental states of others, it can be used in the study of conduct-disorder and callous-unemotional traits.

Other non-standard and advanced measures assess ToM in 'on-line' situations, requiring real-time judgements of information communicated through eye gaze, facial expression, vocal intonation and body movements (Sprung, 2010). Especially sensitive to implicit non-linguistic ToM is the Reading the Mind in the Eyes Test (RMET; Baron-Cohen *et al.*, 2001), which requires the young person to infer another person's mental states from a photograph of only their eye region. It has been used with children of various ages as well as with adults (see Figure 3.1).

In contrast to early research in mentalizing, which addresses the question of whether children are able to understand others' thoughts, later studies have looked into children's *misperception* of the thoughts, feelings and

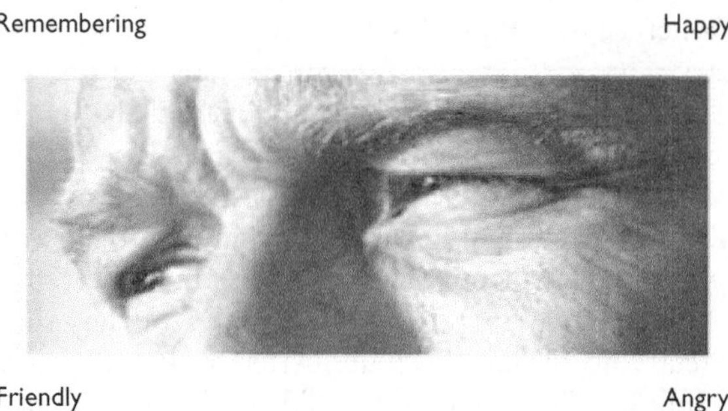

Figure 3.1 An example of the Reading the Mind in the Eyes Test (RMET). Copyright © Simon Baron Cohen, reproduced with kind permission

intentions of others (e.g. O'Connor & Hirsch, 1999). A pioneering task of *distorted* mentalizing in children was developed by Sharp *et al.* (2006). In this task, children are each presented with vignettes containing potentially distressing social scenarios, drawing from themes that may cause unhappiness or distress by depicting emotional and/or physical hurt and social conflict. For example, one story reads: 'One day Peter went to school and during break he went out to the playground. A lot of other kids went out to the playground too, but Peter was the only one sitting alone by the tree. Nobody was sitting or playing with him. Imagine you are Peter. If you were, what do you think the other kids would be thinking about you?'

Children are presented with three response options reflecting one of three mutually exclusive categories: (1) an unrealistic and positive bias with strong self-reference (*They would think I'm cool not to play silly games with the rest of the kids*); (2) a negative bias with strong self-reference (*They would think nobody likes me*); or (3) a neutral/rational/adaptive option devoid of a global, internal and stable self-attribution (*They would think I'm just sitting down to have a think and a rest*). Interestingly, an overly positive mentalizing style in this task was predictive of conduct problems (Sharp *et al.*, 2009).

Various measures have also been developed to assess affective understanding in school-age children. The Kusche's Affective Interview-Revised (KAI-R; Kusche *et al.*, 1988) is one of the most widely used measures. The KAI-R was developed with input from psychodynamic clinical researchers to assess children's emotional understanding at both an experiential and a meta-cognitive level and probes a wide range of affective states. It has been used as an outcome measure in studies showing that school-based programmes promoting emotional understanding can reduce aggression and conduct difficulties. In addition, it has been used to demonstrate that cognitive behavioural treatments focused on increasing emotional understanding are effective for the treatment of anxiety disorders in children (Southam-Gerow & Kendall, 2000).

A number of other promising new measures have been developed to capture important aspects of mentalizing. The Test of Emotional Comprehension (TEC; Pons & Harris, 2005) is of interest because it covers a relatively wide age range (6–12), and because it assesses both affective understanding and ToM. This measure is useful because it has a picture-based multiple choice format that makes scoring relatively easy and relies less on expressive language capacities than many other tests. In spite of its considerable strengths it is probably a test better suited for developmental research rather than therapy outcome studies, unless the therapy under investigation aims to develop the type of generic capacities that are assessed by this test. Also worth noting is the interview measure of emotional regulation and emotional understanding developed by Cunningham *et al.* (2009) from the group working on meta-emotion philosophy (Gottman *et al.*, 1996). It uses vignettes of social scenarios to test dimensions of social and emotional understanding that is strongly reminiscent of the Affect Task (Fonagy *et al.*, 2000) that will be presented later in this chapter. Finally, the Children's Emotion Management Scale of Sadness and Anger (CEMS; Shipman & Zeman, 2001) is another very promising questionnaire measure that makes it possible to assess this very important dimension of children's affective understanding.

Amazing teens: measuring mentalization in adolescents

Recent research has indicated that the marked neural plasticity in the adolescent brain may be implicated in significant improvements in social cognition, which continues to develop well into teens and early twenties (Blakemore, 2008). Along with changes in the neural architecture of mentalizing regions, important changes in self-definition and social relationships present significant challenges as adolescents require advanced mentalizing. Existing measures used with adolescents include, among others, advanced ToM measures, self-reports, vignette-based measures and scales derived from projective assessments. Examples of each type are given below.

Advanced ToM measures have used, for example, visual jokes (cartoons) which require the participants to attribute either false belief or ignorance to one or more of the characters in the picture in order to comprehend the meaning of the joke (Gallagher *et al.*, 2000). Others have used animated objects, such as triangles (e.g. Abell *et al.*, 2000), moving in a self-propelled fashion and interacting in complex ways. Participants in such tests are asked to provide verbal descriptions of the clips, and each respondent's tendency to attribute mental states is assessed by analysing the amount of mental state language used in the descriptions.

In an effort to approximate the demands of everyday life on social cognition, advanced tests have been developed using video footage, such as the Child and Adolescent Social Perception Scale (CASPS; Magill-Evans *et al.*, 1995) and the Movie for the Assessment of Social Cognition (MASC; Dziobek *et al.*, 2006). The former test consists of short videotaped scenes from which the verbal content was removed so that participants could focus on the non-verbal cues. The MASC, on the other hand, uses classical social cognition concepts such as false belief, faux pas, metaphor, or sarcasm to allow for a broad range of mental states to be displayed both verbally and non-verbally (see Chapter 2 for an example).

A few self-report measures have also been developed to assess various aspects of mentalizing. The Basic Empathy Scale (BES; Jolliffe & Farrington, 2006), for example, assesses cognitive and affective empathy. The Reflective Functioning Questionnaire-Adolescent (RFQ-A) was originally developed to follow the principles of the RF scale of the Adult Attachment Interview, for use in adult samples (Fonagy & Ghinai, 2007), and was adapted (Sharp *et al.*, 2009) for use with adolescents by simplifying items to be more developmentally appropriate. The RFQ-A contains both polar scoring items, e.g. '*I'm often curious about the meaning behind others' actions*' and central scoring items, which elicit a balanced mentalizing perspective, whereby participants must recognize that they can know something, but not everything about a person, e.g. '*I can tell how someone is feeling by looking in their eyes*'.

Several vignette-based measures have been also developed to examine various aspects of mentalizing. For instance, the Adolescent Levels of Emotional Awareness Scale (ALEAS; Pratt, 2006) is a scenario-based measure which assesses the participant's ability to provide differentiated and complex descriptions of emotional experience in relation to the self and other people. Respondents are asked to describe in writing how they would feel and how they think the other person would feel in each of the situations, constructed to elicit emotional responses, which can be expressed with varying levels of complexity.

Using a vignette-based, semi-structured interview, O'Connor and Hirsch (1999) assessed 12–14-year-old students' understanding and attributions of mental states of their most and least liked teachers. Students were presented with six situations derived from common school experiences (e.g. 'the student's name was put on the board by the teacher', 'the student was not called on by the teacher even though she or he had her or his hand up', etc.). Following the presentation of each situation, students were asked six questions: Why did this happen? What does the teacher think? What does the teacher feel? What does the student think? What does the student feel? What happens next? Student responses were coded using a system developed for this (O'Connor & Hirsch, 1999), and results indicated that there were significant intra-individual differences in adolescents' mentalizing, which could be predicted from the affective quality of the relationship with each teacher.

More projective measures have been also used to assess mentalization. The Social Cognition and Object Relation Scale (SCORS; Westen *et al.*, 1985, 1990), for instance, was developed to analyse Thematic Apperception Test (TAT) narratives. This is a test that requires the respondent to make up a story based on their personal response to a series of line drawings. Two subscales from the SCORS have been used to measure the domain of mentalization (Rothschild-Yakar *et al.*, 2010), namely: (a) the Complexity of Representations subscale, which measures the degree to which the participant clearly differentiates between the perspectives of the self and others, and the participant's ability to integrate both positive and negative attributes of the self and others; (b) the Understanding Social Causality subscale, which measures the degree to which attributions regarding actions performed by people in the narrative are logical, accurate and psychologically minded.

Integrating cognitive and affective aspects in the measurement of mentalization in middle childhood and adolescence

Although not comprehensive, the above overview highlights that as the construct of ToM and its false belief paradigm were limited to specific tasks and age groups, new measures were developed to capture the developmental progression of ToM and mentalization beyond the prediction of action. These newer measures all aimed to capture the subtleties in the mentalizing abilities of older children in areas that went beyond the original focus on false beliefs.

Nevertheless, most advanced tests mentioned above still have a cognitive focus. Even among those tests assessing an individual's ability to correctly attribute an affective mental state (e.g. '*sad*') to another person, few tests have measured the capacity to infer mental content from the emotion (e.g. '*sadness from saying goodbye*'). Existing tests have relatively neglected the development of the mental processes underlying children's capacity to interpret affective and interpersonal experiences based on their own mental states as well as those of others. Whereas ToM may underemphasize the role that one's social world has in tempering one's ability to represent mental states, mentalization theory has highlighted the significance of social experiences and relationships, particularly those of the child in relation to the parents, in facilitating expression of the capacity for mental representation, above all the representation of intentional states (Ensink, 2003).

Responding to the shortage of age appropriate measures of complex mentalizing abilities in primary-school-age children and adolescents, three measures were developed with our colleagues at University College London and the Anna Freud Centre; they are presented below.

Assessing affective understanding in primary-school-aged children: the Affect Task

The Affect Task (AT; Fonagy *et al.*, 2000) was designed to obtain an objective measure of children's affective understanding, as assessed in the context of a semi-structured interview. It is an adaptation of a preschool version that focuses specifically on the ability to consider mixed and multiple emotions (Steele *et al.*, 1999). This contrasts with the wider focus and more complex coding system of the AT developed for primary-school children (Ensink, 2003) described below.

The AT allows for the systematic differentiation between different levels of sophistication in affective understanding in interpersonal contexts and assesses five dimensions of affective understanding that have been identified by the empirical literature as critical:

1 *Accuracy*: the ability to identify which affects are likely to result given emotion evoking situations.
2 *Justification*: the ability to provide justifications and narratives which show understanding of the causal links between contexts and feelings.
3 *Impact*: the understanding of how feelings change.
4 *Internal/external*: the ability to understand that feelings might be dissembled and that there is a variety of reasons explaining why the feelings shown on the outside might be different from those on the inside.
5 *Challenge*: the ability to imagine and understand that someone else may have a reaction very different from one's own reaction, or a reaction that is not common (Ensink, 2003).

The AT uses line drawings of children portrayed in six emotionally charged everyday situations that were selected because they are familiar to school-age children and because these situations commonly elicit a range of emotions. In each of these drawings there is a central affective theme: bullying, being selected to be captain, being left out, being naughty at the expense of another child, being punished or being in an embarrassing situation. For example, story one is about a bully who pushes over a younger child in front of his or her friends in the school playground (see Figure 3.2).

The AT has an introductory component which is not scored and which introduces the child to line drawings of faces depicting nine different emotional expressions ranging from happy to shocked; these were derived from Ekman *et al.* (1972). The child is asked to identify the different emotions in order to familiarize him or her with the different faces and with

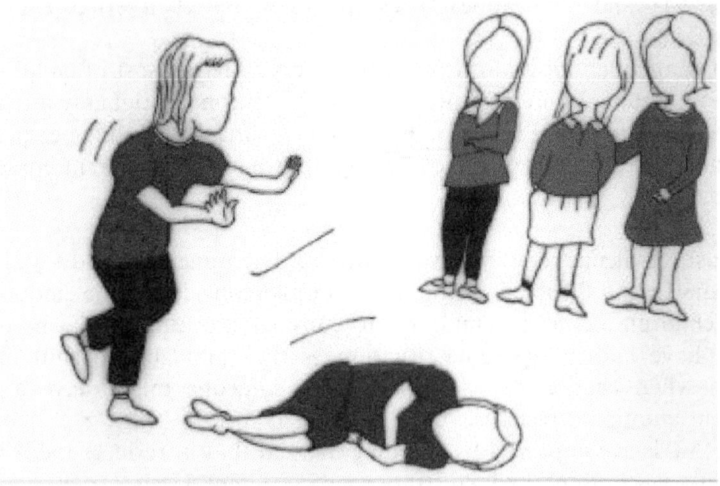

Figure 3.2 An example of an Affect Task card

the idea that each face is meant to represent a different mental state. The same nine faces are then used in acetate form for the next part of the task. In the second and central component of the AT, the child is shown the six cartoon drawings, in which the facial expressions of the characters are blanked out. The interviewer then reads and animates a short script that accompanies each picture. Parallel versions of the six scenarios and accompanying cartoons with boy and girl protagonists are used depending on the gender of the child being interviewed.

After each narrative, the child is invited to choose the appropriate acetate faces to show how all the children in the story might be feeling, using as many faces, or feelings, for each of the characters as he or she may want. Following this, the child is asked:

1 to name all the feelings (used to rate accuracy of the identification of affects)
2 why the characters may be feeling that way (used to rate the capacity to justify and provide a plausible, well-motivated explanation or narrative which explains the different emotional reactions)
3 what happens to the feeling (used to rate the child's knowledge of the fact that the impact of emotions changes over time and his knowledge of the fact that people use specific strategies to reduce the impact of negative feelings)
4 whether the character could be feeling something different on the inside than he is showing on the outside, and then to explain why (used to rate the child's understanding that feelings may be hidden for different

reasons and that appearances may not reflect internal emotional experience)

5 to imagine and explain why another 'very different sort of child' might have a quite different response to the one they had originally attributed to the character (used to rate the child's capacity to shift perspectives and consider why someone else might have a quite different emotional reaction).

This last 'challenge' question was added to determine the child's ability to be recursive and flexible in thinking about and considering the emotions of other children, i.e. is the child able to consider the feelings that he or she would have had in the same situation, is the child able to shift mental frames when challenged to consider why someone might have a quite different emotional response, etc. (Ensink, 2003).

The AT is accompanied by a coding manual that introduces the AT and contains descriptions and illustrations of different levels for each of the abilities that are assessed. The coding system provides a systematic approach to scoring children's responses and uses a hierarchical approach that differentiates between five levels of mentalization on the basis of elaboration and complexity. The approach used to rate responses to the Accuracy and Justification questions has been outlined by Ensink (2003).

The psychometric properties of the AT were assessed in a sample of 175 children aged 5–11, 65 of whom were recruited from schools and 110 from referrals to Child and Adolescent Mental Health Services (CAMHS) in London (Ensink, 2003). In sum, the study results supported the use of the AT as a reliable and valid method for assessing affective understanding in primary-school-age children. In addition, poor affective understanding was associated with depression and externalization disorder, and the ability to understand the causes of emotions in interpersonal terms was associated with attachment security.

Assessing mentalization in the context of attachment relationships: the Child Reflective Functioning Scale

The Child Reflective Functioning Scale (CRFS; Ensink, 2003) was adapted from the Adult Reflective Functioning Scale (ARFS; Fonagy *et al.*, 1998) and was developed to assess the extent to which primary-school children aged 8 to 11 consider themselves and their significant relationships in mental state terms. The CRFS was designed for use with the Child Attachment Interview (CAI; Target *et al.*, 2000), in parallel with the use of the ARFS on Adult Attachment Interview narratives, although the CRFS was found to require a somewhat different scoring procedure. Shmueli-Goetz and colleagues (2008), using the CAI, confirmed that primary-school-age children can respond in a meaningful manner to direct questions about themselves, their attachment relationships and situations of conflict. Like the ARFS, the CRFS can be applied to data obtained using other interviews, e.g. regarding relationships with peers and close friends.

The important caveat here is that reflective functioning, like attachment, is revealed in the context of speaking about oneself and one's close relationships (Fonagy & Target, 2003); thus it is expected that it will be most evident in the context of being asked to describe specific incidents which reveal something about the self, interpersonal interactions and affective reactions. In fact, the most elaborate mentalization is commonly shown in efforts to explain interpersonally difficult incidents, e.g. involving conflict or confusing behaviour. These descriptions require a process of retrieval of specific events and narratives, and these episodic or autobiographical memories are expected to provide a good indicator of the child's 'working knowledge' of mental states and of both intrapersonal and interpersonal thinking (Ensink, 2003). These memories are expected to reflect an ability quite different from that demonstrated when the child describes relationships in general terms; in the latter case, intellectual ability is expected to play a greater role. In this respect, the structure of the adult and child attachment interviews, which ask specifically for examples illustrating why a particular adjective was chosen to describe the self or a close relationship, is ideal for assessing reflective functioning (Ensink, 2003).

The CRFS coding system is designed so that raters can make an objective assessment of children's ability to provide mentalizing accounts of themselves, their key attachment relationships and their context. The raters assess descriptions that children provide of specific memories or events to illustrate key qualities of themselves and their relationships. The manual (Ensink, 2003) selected from the CAI the following questions for RF rating:

1 the three "self-description" questions
2 the "self upset" question
3 the three "relationship with mother" questions
4 the "mother cross/upset" question
5 the "relationship with father" question
6 the "father cross/upset" question
7 the "parents argue" question.

The rationale for proposing this particular set of questions was that it is applicable to all children, and includes questions about the self, relationships and affectively charged situations.

The final coding ranges from 1–9, with 1 being equal to narratives that contain no use of psychological explanation, and 9 representing elaborated psychological accounts of relationship experiences.

The revised CRFS was used to code the CAI data of a sample of 61 children aged 8–11, all recruited from referrals to CAMHS in London

(Ensink, 2003). In sum, the study results confirmed that the psychometric properties of the CRFS were robust; and children's reflective functioning as measured by the CRFS was predicted by age and attachment, and not by intelligence. It was concluded both that it is possible to assess reflective functioning reliably in relatively young children and that reflective functioning is an ability closely linked to attachment (Ensink, 2003). The CRFS has subsequently been used in a study of sexually abused children in Québec, Canada (Ensink *et al.*, submitted) and the results of this study provide further evidence of the validity of the CRFS.

Mad, sad, bad or a cool lad? The Mentalizing Stories for Adolescents (MSA)

While the CRFS importantly measures cognitive processes related to mentalization in an attachment context, it is difficult to employ in large-scale research or use routinely in clinical settings. The Mentalizing Stories for Adolescents (MSA) was developed in order to assess the quality of mental state understanding in a contextually and affectively embedded form using a multiple-choice format.

The original open-ended version of the MSA has been described in detail elsewhere (Vrouva & Fonagy, 2009). In summary, it consists of 20 vignettes in which a negative interaction takes place between the protagonist and another person, who is usually the protagonist's friend, or classmate, or sibling, or parent. The interactions are not entirely imaginary or highly fictional, but describe adolescence-relevant everyday situations. Each situation was constructed to elicit feelings such as sadness, anger, disappointment, or jealousy in the protagonist, who does or says something as a result of this emotional state. After reading each vignette, respondents are asked to answer briefly, with a few sentences, why the central character behaved in the story as they did.

Accordingly, the MSA assesses mentalizing that is controlled/explicit, namely that is conscious, verbal, and requires attention, awareness and effort. It envisions the mind of another (the protagonist in each story), and focuses on mental interiors (internal based), directly considering feelings, thoughts and experiences, rather than on physical and visible features. The MSA is considered to capture elements of both affective and cognitive mentalization, which only in combination would generate genuine social understanding, what has been termed mentalized affectivity or 'the feeling of feeling' (Fonagy *et al.*, 2002).

Despite its promising psychometric properties, the open-ended version of the MSA was rather cumbersome and heavily dependent on written communication and the participants' willingness to elaborate in this form. Therefore subsequent multiple-choice versions were administered to a total of 439 primary and secondary school students; the properties of these earlier versions are available from the first author on request. Below we describe the final (and most successful) multiple-choice version.

For each story of the MSA, four options were selected on the basis of a formal categorization, allowing the new multiple-choice format to differentiate three different types of mistakes that reflect:

a a physical reality justification with an evasive, dismissive quality, which is plausible but fails to acknowledge the main conflict presented in the story and provides instead a non-mental, situational justification
b inaccurate or excessive mentalizing directed towards others; the protagonist's attributions reflect exaggerated blaming of the other person in the story
c inaccurate or excessive mentalizing directed towards the self; the protagonist's attributions are self-blaming or self-diminishing.

These three types of incorrect answers were used as models to construct distractor answers. Each stem also contains an accurate mentalizing justification (correct option). In addition, the MSA contains two control stories, which do not involve mental states and would permit some certainty regarding a participant's reading comprehension or attention to the task. There is also an image next to each story to facilitate comprehension. An example MSA item is presented below:

> Oliver's maths teacher has just announced the results of the exam. Oliver did very well. At home in the evening, he says to his father: 'I got the third highest mark in the class.' His father says: 'Hmm, first is always better than third.' Oliver leaves the room quickly and spends the rest of the evening in his bedroom alone.
>
> *Q*: Why do you think Oliver might have done this?
>
> (a) Oliver wants to finish his coursework early and watch TV.
> (b) Oliver is annoyed with his father for trying to humiliate and depress him.
> (c) Oliver is sad; he hoped that his father would have congratulated him.
> (d) Oliver regrets that he didn't study harder to make his father happy.

The first option (a) represents a physical reality justification with an evasive, dismissive quality. The second option (b) represents inaccurate or excessive mentalizing directed towards others, whereas the fourth (d) represents inaccurate or excessive mentalizing directed towards the self. The third option (c) is the correct answer (accurate mentalizing justification).

This latest version of the MSA was administered to an adolescent (n=116) and a young adult (n=58) group. In both groups, females scored on average higher than males, which is in agreement with the findings of studies suggesting a female advantage on various aspects of social cognition. Older adolescents did better at the MSA, and this association was significant only in females. Moreover, the young adult group's MSA score was higher than the adolescent group's score. The psychometric properties of the MSA were robust in this study and were replicated in a study of 49 predominantly disadvantaged, inner-city North American adolescents (Rutherford *et al.*, submitted).

In conclusion, the MSA was developed in an attempt to strike a balance between projective, open-ended tasks and more forced-choice ability measures. As the incorrect options are cognitively plausible but reflect an incongruent affective valence, the task taps the more complex mental state understanding that is dependent on young people's *interpretations* of the same information given in each story. Another significant feature of the MSA is that it was developed for use with young people and is composed of situations consistent with the adolescent perspective. However, the degree to which different participants could relate to the content of different stories is unknown.

Challenges and opportunities in measuring mentalization

In this chapter, we have summarized the different constructs and the measures that index various aspects of mentalization in children and young people. Some key considerations affecting all such measurement are gathered together below.

How to access mentalization capacities?

We saw that the various measures can be classified according to the age they are pitched at, the method used to present the stimuli and collect the data (e.g. observation, interview, self-report, vignettes, video footage, animated shapes, etc.), and most importantly, the type of mentalization that each task is aimed at assessing (e.g. external: face processing tasks; cognitive: belief-desire reasoning tasks; attachment-relevant: CRFS, etc.). We also saw that the coding system used in some measures of mentalization can be complex and require significant ability and skill at the level of interpretation. On the other hand, tests that do not require individual administration and scoring may also be limited in that some significant dimensions of mentalization are inherently interpersonal and can therefore be best elicited and evaluated within an interpersonal, one-to-one interview framework.

In studying older children, it is apparent that traditional methods have been extended and alternative methods and conceptualizations have been employed to distinguish individual differences. The application of new technologies has enabled us to use computerized tasks, to include assessment of reaction times, to detect the brain areas activated during certain mentalizing tasks, etc. Such technological advances have taken place in parallel with developments in the conceptualization of mentalization and the increased understanding that mentalization is a multifaceted ability which cannot be fully captured by a single task.

Assessing mentalization in preschoolers and toddlers

In contrast to the growing range of potential measures for assessing mentalization in school-aged children and adolescents, the options for assessing mentalization in preschoolers are much more limited. At this stage most validated experimental assessments either focus quite narrowly on ToM capacities or on socio-emotional understanding of a more general type. These measures may be useful to identify children with overt deficits in mentalization, but they have serious limitations when it comes to assessing more nuanced mentalization difficulties in children. New and innovative paradigms for assessing the mentalization capacities of preschoolers, especially mentalization capacities that have more personal relevance, need to be developed. The assessment of preschoolers' mentalization capacities through play provides a potentially promising avenue for the assessment of children's mentalization. Consistent with Fonagy and Target's theoretical proposals regarding the importance of play as a precursor of reflective function, recent research suggests that mentalization can be reliably measured in children's free play and predicts later performance on the CRFS (Tessier *et al.*, 2009).

Self vs. other focus

Differences in mentalizing about self and others have received relatively little attention, although most authors agree that similarities and distinctions between these two types of mentalization and their developmental progression is critical to explaining the origins of mentalizing (Happé, 2003). The vast majority of tasks assess mentalization in relation to others and very few attempts have been made to operationalize the understanding children have of themselves, their own thought processes and especially their awareness of the mental and behavioural strategies that they use when they are confronted with affects such as sadness and anger. Shipman and Zeman (2001) have piloted some very promising interviews and self-report measures to assess children's emotional management strategies, but further work in this area is needed. At this point we still know comparatively little about the development of children's capacity to self-define, whether this can be regarded as a good indicator of identity and whether this is related to psychosocial adaptation. Clinically, this is a very significant domain as some children's ability to report on their internalizing symptoms may be limited because of their insufficient ability to reflect on their own mental states (see Chapter 2 and also Sprung, 2010).

The role of context

We also saw that mentalization is expected to vary depending on the relationship context in question, or the intensity of affect, and that it might be sensitive to the context or timing of the assessment (Choi-Kain & Gunderson, 2008). Research on intra-individual differences in mentalizing is required to integrate research on relationships and social cognition and to explore what inhibits or promotes the ability or motivation to use mentalization in a particular relationship (O'Connor & Hirsch, 1999). Such studies may use instruments that measure mentalization with regard to a specific relationship (e.g. favourite vs. least favourite teacher), but they may also use experimental paradigms in which mentalization is assessed in a given emotional context.

Reflecting on pleasant or unpleasant states of mind

It is also important to consider the valence of mental states presented in the various tests. Equal awareness of mental states with different valence (positive and negative) is important for healthy psychological functioning and an imbalance has been linked to various clinical conditions (see Chapter 2 and Sprung, 2010). Measures that tap affective understanding should therefore enable us to detect preoccupation with either negative or positive mental states in self and others and its potential impact on how children relate to others as well as to themselves.

Mentalization in real life

It is important to recognize that no measure can ever completely capture the reality and dynamism of people's everyday lives and that on-line, 'hot' mentalization is particularly hard to assess. Both naturalistic and experimental methods are important to consider for this reason. Experiments based in game theoretic paradigms, which have been widely used in the economic literature, may capture the on-line component of mentalization exactly because they simulate real-world interpersonal interactions in which the extent to which one is able to read social signals has implications for the outcome of the interaction. Despite such admirable paradigms, it may be still impossible to assess on-line mentalization in some contexts. For example, we may hypothesize that mentalization drops in distressing contexts. However, such contexts may not lend themselves to direct observation for ethical and practical reasons.

Mentalizing shown indirectly

Another important consideration is that although the capacity to mentalize may be mostly apparent in verbal behaviour, it also manifests itself in more implicit ways. For instance, a parent who remains silent in the face of their adolescent's aggressive outburst and who waits for the storm to pass maybe applying mentalization much more efficiently than another parent who in the heat of the moment accurately, yet rather unhelpfully, comments on their child's mental states and questions what triggered them. Therefore measures need to take into account this indirect yet very significant aspect of mentalization which goes one step further in that it requires the application of mental state understanding in real-world social behaviour.

Important influences moderating or limiting task performance

Beyond these general measurement issues, several factors are known to influence the sensitivity of assessments of children's abilities. Children may have difficulty understanding the instructions of the task, maintaining attention and establishing rapport and motivation (Ensink, 2003). This is a particularly important consideration when using experimental paradigms to assess mentalization in preschoolers where temperamental and maturational factors may make it challenging for the examiner to fully engage the child and focus their attention on the task. For example, some preschoolers with highly sociable and surgent temperaments may become over-excited and distracted in the experimental situation when presented with attractive puppets. They may be so intent on engaging the interviewer in play that this may interfere with the capacity to observe their real abilities with regard to emotional understanding. Other difficulties, such as attention deficit hyperactivity disorder (ADHD), depression, and learning or sensory disabilities may also affect performance and result in an underestimation of mentalization. However, it is reasonable to expect that IQ shares a considerable degree of variance with mentalizing, as attaining high levels of mentalizing is a quite complex task (Thomas & Maio, 2008).

Hartmann (1992) also points out that because of significant developmental changes, scores on a particular measure may be a valid indicator of ability at a given age, but may primarily reflect motivation at an older age. This is particularly relevant when tests are not challenging enough for certain age groups. On the other hand, tasks that tap into newly emerging abilities may also be unreliable, as assessing transient performance levels may lead to lower reliability in measurement (Ensink, 2003).

Further consideration also needs to be given to the assessment of children from different cultural and linguistic backgrounds (Ensink, 2003), as different norms regarding social interactions and talking about emotions and relationships across generations are expected to affect the performance of children from different cultures on various measures of social understanding. In addition, most measures require that children have more than a working knowledge of the language used in the task, and children tested in a second language may thus appear to function at a much lower level than when they use their mother tongue (Ensink, 2003). Further research is needed to determine the impact of language abilities on mentalization, as well as the cross-cultural application of the various tests.

Reflections on using mentalization measures in outcome research

The mentalization measures that have been presented have evident value in the context of research documenting the development of children's mentalization capacities, as well as in investigating the relationship between mentalization and psychopathology. A key question however concerns their potential usefulness as psychotherapy outcome measures. Measures have to be very carefully chosen and often specially adapted to assess the very specific domains of mentalization where therapy is most likely to produce changes. For example, if the therapy aims to increase understanding of the conflicts that underlie anxiety states, measures that specifically target mentalization in this area will be most effective in demonstrating the changes resulting from therapy. Unless an explicit aim of therapy is to facilitate the development of mentalization capacities more broadly, the use of more general measures of mentalization may fail to detect important therapeutic achievements.

Conclusion

This chapter has offered an introduction to the various measurement challenges of assessing mentalization in children and young people. As mental states are not obvious, but potentially at odds with overt behaviour or external reality (Wellman & Liu, 2004), measuring the complex ability of understanding mental states in developmental periods – that vary in complexity and domain relevance – is a demanding process. Since mentalization is a multifaceted process that undergoes changes throughout development, sequences of mentalization growth may have different trajectories as children are called to negotiate their increasingly complex social world (Bosacki & Astington, 1999). There is much more to be learnt about mentalizing across development beyond labelling mental states in self and others. We hope that measures such as the CRFS, the AT and the MSA will be updated as we learn more about the construct and its developmental vicissitudes.

References

Abell, F., Happé, F., & Frith, U. (2000). Do triangles play tricks? Attribution of mental states to animated shapes in normal and abnormal development. *Journal of Cognitive Development*, 15, 1–20.

Allen, J. G. (2003). Mentalizing. *Bulletin of the Menninger Clinic*, 67(2), 91–112.

Baron-Cohen, S., O'Riordan, M., Stone, V., Jones, R., & Plaisted, K. (1999). Recognition of faux pas by normally developing children and children with Asperger syndrome or high-functioning autism. *Journal of Autism and Developmental Disorders*, 29, 407–418.

Baron-Cohen, S., Wheelwright, S., Scahill, V., Lawson, J., & Spong, A. (2001). Are intuitive physics and intuitive psychology independent? A test with children with Asperger syndrome. *Journal of Developmental and Learning Disorders*, 5, 47–78.

Blakemore, S. J. (2008). The social brain in adolescence. *Nature Reviews Neuroscience*, 9(4), 267–277.

Bosacki, S., & Astington, J. W. (1999). Theory of mind in preadolescence: Relations between social understanding and social competence. *Social Development*, 8, 237–255.

Choi-Kain, L. W., & Gunderson, J. G. (2008). Mentalization: Ontogeny, assessment, and application in the treatment of borderline personality disorder. *American Journal of Psychiatry*, 165(9), 1127–1135.

Cunningham, J. N., Kliewer, W., & Garner, P. (2009). Emotion socialization, child emotion understanding and regulation, and adjustment in urban African American families: Differential associations across child gender. *Development and Psychopathology*, 21, 261–283.

Denham, S. A. (1986). Social cognition, prosocial behavior, and emotion in preschoolers: Contextual validation. *Child Development*, 57, 194–201.

Denham, S. A. (2006). Social-emotional competence as support for school readiness: What is it and how do we assess it? *Early Education and Development*, 17(1), 57–89.

Dennett, D. C. (1987). *The intentional stance*. Cambridge, MA: MIT Press.

Dunn, J., Brown, J., & Beardsall, L. (1991). Family talk about feeling states and children's later understanding of others' emotions. *Developmental Psychology*, 27, 448–455.

Dziobek, I., Fleck, S., Kalbe, E., Rogers, K., Hassenstab, J., Brand, M., *et al.* (2006). Introducing MASC: A movie for the assessment of social cognition. *Journal of Autism and Developmental Disorders*, 36(5), 623–636.

Ekman, P., Friesen, W. V., & Ellsworth, P. (1972). *Emotion in the human face*. New York: Pergamon Press.

Ensink, K. (2003). Assessing theory of mind, affective understanding and reflective functioning in primary school-aged children. Unpublished doctoral dissertation. London: University College London.

Ensink, K., Normandin, L., Sabourin, S., Fonagy, P., & Target, M. (submitted).

Mentalisation in middle-childhood: An initial study of the validity of the Child Reflective Functioning Scale.

Flavell, J. H., Green, F.L., & Flavell, E.R. (2000). Development of children's awareness of their own thoughts. *Journal of Cognition & Development*, 1, 1–12.

Fonagy, P., & Target, M. (2003). *Psychoanalytic theories: perspectives from developmental psychopathology*. New York: Brunner-Routledge.

Fonagy, P., & Ghinai, R. (2007). A self-report measure of mentalizing: Development and preliminary test of the reliability and validity of the Reflective Function Questionnaire (RFQ). Unpublished manuscript. London: University College London.

Fonagy, P., & Luyten, P. (2009). A developmental, mentalization-based approach to the understanding and treatment of borderline personality disorder. *Development and Psychopathology*, 21(4), 1355–1381.

Fonagy, P., Gergely, G., Jurist, E., & Target, M. (2002). *Affect regulation, mentalization and the development of the self.* New York: Other Press.

Fonagy, P., Target, M., Steele, H., & Steele, M. (1998). *Reflective-functioning manual, version 5.0, for application to Adult Attachment Interviews.* London: University College London.

Fonagy, P., Target, M., & Ensink, K. (2000). *The affect task: Unpublished measure and coding manual.* London: Anna Freud Centre.

Gallagher, H. L., Happé, F., Brunswick, N., Fletcher, P. C., Frith, U., & Frith, C. D. (2000). Reading the mind in cartoons and stories: An fMRI study of 'theory of mind' in verbal and nonverbal tasks. *Neuropsychologia*, 38, 11–21.

Gergely, G., Nadasdy, Z., Csibra, G., & Biro, S. (1995). Taking the intentional stance at 12 months of age. *Cognition*, 56, 165–193.

Gottman, J. M., Katz, L. F., & Hooven, C. (1996). Parental meta-emotion philosophy and the emotional life of families: Theoretical models and preliminary data. *Journal of Family Psychology*, 10(3), 243–268.

Happé, F. (1994). An advanced test of theory of mind: Understanding of story characters' thoughts and feelings by able autistic, mentally handicapped, and normal children and adults. *Journal of Autism and Developmental Disorders*, 24, 129–154.

Happé, F. (2003). Theory of mind and the self. *Annals of the New York Academy of Sciences*, 1001, 134–144.

Hartmann, D. P. (1992). Design, measurement, and analysis: Technical issues in developmental research. In M. H. Bornstein & M. H. Lamb (Eds.), *Developmental psychology: An advanced textbook* (3rd ed., pp. 59–151). Hillsdale, NJ: Lawrence Erlbaum Associates, Inc.

Jolliffe, D., & Farrington, D. P. (2006). The development and validation of the basic empathy scale. *Journal of Adolescence*, 29, 589–611.

Kusche, C. A., Beilke, R. L., & Greenberg, M. T. (1988). Kusche Affective Interview-Revised. Unpublished measure. Washington, WA: University of Washington, Seattle.

Magill-Evans, J., Koning, C., Cameron-Sadava, A., & Manyk, K. (1995). The Child and Adolescent Social Perception measure. *Journal of Nonverbal Behavior*, 19, 151–169.

Measelle, J. R., Ablow, J. C., Cowan, P. A., & Cowan, C. P. (1998). Assessing young children's views of their academic, social, and emotional lives: An evaluation of the self-perception scales of the Berkeley Puppet Interview. *Child Development*, 69(6), 1556–1576.

O'Connor, T., & Hirsch, N. (1999). Intra-individual differences and relationship-specicity of mentalising in early adolescence. *Social Development*, 8, 256–274.

Pons, F., & Harris, P. L. (2005). Longitudinal change and longitudinal stability of individual differences in children's emotion understanding. *Cognition and Emotion*, 19(8), 1158–1174.

Pratt, B. M. (2006). Emotional intelligence and the emotional brain: A battery of tests of ability applied with high school students and adolescents with high-functioning autistic spectrum disorders. Unpublished doctoral dissertation: Sydney: University of Sydney.

Rogers, J. S. C., Viding, E., Blair, R. J. R., Frith, U., & Happé, F. (2006). Autism spectrum disorder and psychopathy: Shared cognitive underpinnings or double hit? *Psychological Medicine*, 36, 1789–1798.

Rothschild-Yakar, L., Levy-Shiff, R., Fridman-Balaban, R., Gur, E., & Stein, D. (2010). Mentalization and relationships with parents as predictors of eating disordered behavior. *Journal of Nervous and Mental Disorders*, 198(7), 501–507.

Rutherford, J. V., Wareham, J. D., Vrouva, I., Mayes, L. C., Fonagy, P., & Potenza, M. (submitted). Sex differences in adolescent mentalization and its relationship to theory of mind and language functioning. Manuscript under review.

Sharp, C., & Fonagy, P. (2008). The parent's capacity to treat the child as a psychological agent: Constructs, measures and implications for developmental psychopathology. *Social Development*, 17(3), 737–754.

Sharp, C., Fonagy, P., & Goodyer, I. M. (2006). Imagining your child's mind: Psychosocial adjustment and mothers' ability to predict their children's attributional response styles. *British Journal of Developmental Psychology*, 24, 197–214.

Sharp, C., Williams, L. L., Ha, C., Baumgardner, J., Michonski, J., Seals, R., *et al.* (2009). The development of a mentalization-based outcomes and research protocol for an adolescent inpatient unit. *Bulletin of the Menninger Clinic*, 73(4), 311–338.

Shipman, K., & Zeman, J. (2001). Socialization of children's emotion regulation in mother–child dyads: A developmental psychopathology perspective. *Development and Psychopathology*, 13, 317–336.

Shmueli-Goetz, Y., Target, M., Fonagy, P., & Datta, A. (2008). The Child Attachment Interview: A psychometric study of reliability and discriminant validity. *Developmental Psychology*, 44, 939–956.

Southam-Gerow, M. A., & Kendall, P. C. (2000). A preliminary study of the emotion understanding of youth referred for treatment of anxiety disorders. *Journal of Clinical Child Psychology*, 29, 319–327.

Sprung, M. (2010). Clinically relevant measures of children's theory of mind and knowledge about thinking: Focus on other, not standard and advanced measures. *Child and Adolescent Mental Health*, 15(4), 204–216.

Steele, H., & Steele, M. (2005). Understanding and resolving emotional conflict: The London Parent–Child Project. In K. E. Grossmann, K. Grossmann & E. Waters (Eds.), *Attachment from infancy to adulthood* (pp. 137–164). New York: Guilford Press.

Steele, H., Steele, M., Croft, C., & Fonagy, P. (1999). Infant–mother attachment at one year predicts children's understanding of mixed emotions at six years. *Social Development*, 8, 161–174.

Target, M., Fonagy, P., Shmueli-Goetz, Y., Schneider, T., & Datta, A. (2000). Child Attachment Interview (CAI): Coding and classification manual, Version III. Unpublished manuscript. London: University College London.

Target, M., Oandasan, C., L, & Ensink, K. (2001). Child reflective functioning coding manual. Unpublished manuscript. London: University College London.

Tessier, V. P., Rousseau, M.-E., Ensink, K., & Normandin, L. (2009, October). Relationship between play, sexual abuse, and reflective functioning in children. Poster presented at the Society for Psychotherapy Research – Canadian meeting (SPR-CA). Montréal, Canada.

Thomas, G., & Maio, G. R. (2008). Man, I feel like a woman: When and how gender-role motivation helps mind-reading. *Journal of Personality and Social Psychology*, 95(5), 1165–1179.

Vrouva, I. (2010). Self-harming and borderline personality disorder traits in adolescence: The role of attachment relationships and mentalizing. Unpublished doctoral dissertation. London: University College London.

Vrouva, I., & Fonagy, P. (2009). Mind the mind! The Mentalization Stories' Test for Adolescents. *Journal of the American Psychoanalytic Association*, 57(5), 1174–1179.

Wellman, H. M., & Liu, D. (2004). Scaling of theory-of-mind tasks. *Child Development*, 75(2), 523–541.

Westen, D., Lohr, N., Silk, K., & Kerber, K. (1985). Measuring object relations and social cognition using the TAT: Scoring manual. Unpublished manuscript. Michigan, MI: University of Michigan.

Westen, D., Lohr, N., Silk, K. R., & Kerber, K. (1990). Object relations and social cognition in borderlines, major depressives, and normals: A thematic apperception test analysis. *Psychological Assessment*, 2(4), 355–364.

Part II

Clinic-based interventions

Chapter 4

Mentalization-based treatment for parents (MBT-P) with borderline personality disorder and their infants

Liesbet Nijssens, Patrick Luyten and Dawn L. Bales

Introduction

The Centre for Psychotherapy Viersprong is a mental health care institute in the Netherlands which specializes in the assessment and treatment of personality disorders. Viersprong also has its own research institute, the Viersprong Institute for Studies on Personality Disorders (VISPD), which aims to facilitate patient-focused, evidence-based and cost-effective care for patients with personality disorders. The Mentalization-Based Treatment (MBT) Unit within Viersprong is dedicated to the treatment of patients with severe personality disorder, in particular patients with borderline personality disorder (BPD) who typically have multiple co-morbid Axis I and Axis II disorders.

Within the unit various versions of MBT are offered, including day-hospital MBT for adult BPD patients (MBT-DH), intensive outpatient MBT for adult BPD patients (MBT-IOP), intensive outpatient MBT for adolescent BPD patients (MBT-A), and MBT for families (MBT-F). We recently started with the implementation of a new variant of MBT, i.e. MBT for Parents (MBT-P), a reflective parenting programme for parents with BPD and their infants. This programme focuses on parenting and the parent–child relationship, in particular in parents with BPD, and aims to improve the parent–child relationship by enhancing the capacity for parental reflective functioning (PRF), i.e. the capacity of the parents to reflect upon their own and their child's internal mental experience (Slade, 2005). In this way, it is also hoped that infant development can be fostered and the probability of the intergenerational transmission of BPD decreased. This chapter reports on the theoretical background, development, structure and intervention principles of MBT-P.

Borderline personality disorder and impairments in mentalizing

According to Fonagy *et al.* (2011), the core features of BPD include: (a) emotional dysregulation (Linehan, 1993; Reisch *et al.*, 2008); (b) high levels of impulsivity (Grootens *et al.*, 2008) leading to self-harm and suicidality (Black, Blum, Pfohl, & Hale, 2004); (c) disturbed interpersonal functioning (Hill *et al.*, 2008). It is a fundamental assumption of the mentalization-based approach to BPD that these symptoms are rooted in impairments in mentalization. Within this view, impairments in mentalization are considered to be closely related to increased stress and arousal, particularly in the context of attachment relationships (Fonagy *et al.*, 2010, 2011). More specifically, BPD patients are thought to be characterized by a low threshold for activation of the attachment system under stress, often reflected by a mixture of attachment hyperactivating and deactivating strategies, leading to impairments in their mentalizing capacities (Fonagy *et al.*, 2011). This sequence typically results first in hyper-mentalization and then in the breakdown of mentalization (Ensink & Mayes, 2010; Fonagy *et al.*, 2011). The disappearance of controlled mentalizing subsequently leads to the re-emergence of non-mentalizing modes, i.e. modes of thinking that antedate the capacity for full mentalization (i.e. psychic equivalence, teleological and extreme pretend mode), which may explain the typical features associated with BPD (Fonagy & Luyten, 2009; see also Chapter 1).

MBT is a treatment programme originally designed for patients with BPD (Bateman & Fonagy, 2004, 2006), which aims to enhance reflective functioning capacities. Following reports of the efficacy of MBT-DH (Bateman & Fonagy, 1999, 2001, 2008) and MBT-IOP (Bateman & Fonagy, 2009), both variants of MBT for BPD were implemented by Viersprong in 2004 and 2008, respectively. A recently completed naturalistic study among 45 BPD patients of MBT-DH largely replicated the results of the Bateman and Fonagy (1999) MBT-DH trial, indicating that MBT can be effectively implemented in an independent treatment institute outside of the UK (Bales *et al.*, in press).

Yet over the past years we came to realize that an increasing number of pregnant women and young parents with BPD features were admitted to Viersprong for treatment. Importantly, we noticed that these patients, despite showing improvements in reflective functioning and clinical measures, evidenced only slight improvements with regard to parental reflective functioning (PRF), i.e. their ability to envision their child in terms of internal mental states (Slade, 2005). For instance, a father of a 13-month-old baby stated that he could not imagine that his excessive alcohol abuse and anger tantrums would have any impact on his little boy: 'It doesn't affect him. And moreover, he is too small to remember it. Maybe in a few years it will have an impact on him, but now?'

Based on similar experiences and the growing realization that mentalizing is to a large extent relationship-specific (Fonagy & Luyten, 2009; Luyten *et al.*, 2009), we came to the conclusion that standard MBT may not sufficiently foster the capacity for PRF, because standard MBT does not have a direct focus on the capacity for reflective functioning in relation to the child. Further, several research findings suggest that children of parents with BPD display deficits in emotion regulation, show sometimes marked distortions in self and other representations, and have a higher prevalence of disorganized attachment patterns, resulting in an increased risk for BPD and other types of psychopathology and problems in psychosocial functioning more generally (Levy *et al.*, 2011; Macfie, 2009; Steele & Siever, 2010). The observation of impaired and distorted PRF in combination with the growing realization of the risk for the intergenerational transmission of psychopathology in parents with BPD was a cause of concern with respect to the development of their children, and became the key impetus for the development of MBT-P. The aims of MBT-P are therefore: (a) to improve parental reflective functioning; (b) in order to improve the quality of parent–child interactions; and (c) in so doing to decrease the risk for the intergenerational transmission of BPD and psychopathology more generally.

The importance of parental reflective functioning

PRF refers to the parent's capacity to reflect upon her own and her child's internal mental experience, to understand behaviour in the light of underlying mental states and intentions (Slade, 2005; Slade *et al.*, 2005a). It has been associated with positive child development and the intergenerational transmission of attachment security (for a review, see Ensink & Mayes, 2010; Fonagy & Target, 2005; Slade, 2005; Sharp & Fonagy, 2008).

Over the past years, similar concepts have been introduced by various research groups. Elizabeth Meins and colleagues, for instance, introduced the concept of maternal mind-mindedness (MMM), which is the proclivity of the parent to treat her infant as an individual with a mind, rather than merely as an infant with needs that must be satisfied (Meins, 1997, 1999). MMM and PRF are both operationalizations of the concept of parental mentalization, with MMM expressing itself in real-life interactions with the child, and PRF expressing itself through the metacognitive representations that the mother holds about her relationship with the child (Sharp & Fonagy, 2008). Interestingly, MMM takes into account the appropriateness of mothers' interactions with their infants (Meins *et al.*, 2001). This makes MMM especially relevant to BPD, as many BPD parents may attribute mental states to their child, but in quite inappropriate ways. For instance, a 19-year-old mother with BPD was enthusiastically playing peek-a-boo with her three-month-old daughter by putting a little blanket on her baby's face and subsequently removing it while saying 'Hi there' in a loud voice. The infant became scared and immediately started crying. The mother did not realize that her little daughter was too young to understand and enjoy this pretend game. More importantly, she then interpreted her infant's crying as an indication on the infant's part that she did not want to play with her.

Because of this, she withdrew from her daughter and left her crying, adding: 'Now she can play by herself', which led to even greater distress.

Substantial evidence indicates that (appropriate) parental mentalization predicts attachment security, adaptive social-cognitive skills, an increased sense of self-efficacy, the development of structures crucial to self and affect regulation, and the mentalizing abilities in offspring (e.g. Arnott & Meins, 2007; Grienenberger *et al.*, 2005; Meins *et al.*, 2002, 2003; Rosenblum *et al.*, 2008; Slade *et al.*, 2005a). By contrast, impairments in PRF have been associated with various forms of psychopathology in the child, from disrupted attachment in infancy and childhood, to a range of personality disorders in adulthood, including BPD (Gottman *et al.*, 1996; Katz & Windecker-Nelson, 2004; Sharp & Fonagy, 2008; Sharp *et al.*, 2006; Slade, 2005).

It is important to note that parental mentalization is not the only determinant of child psychopathology, and should always be considered among a variety of factors, such as child temperament, parental psychopathology, family structure, life events, and genetic predispositions (Sharp & Fonagy, 2008). Nevertheless, the research referenced above suggests that PRF is important enough to be a central focus in the treatment of parents with BPD, particularly because of its purported role in the intergenerational transmission of attachment (Sharp & Fonagy, 2008; Slade, 2005) and the growing evidence that mentalization-based interventions are associated with improvements in PRF (e.g. Sadler *et al.*, 2006; Slade, 2005, 2006; Suchman *et al.*, 2008, 2010).

Existing reflective parenting programmes have as a primary aim the development of a reflective stance in parents, i.e. to engage parents in thinking about their children in terms of their internal experience rather than their behaviour. The Parents First programme (Goyette-Ewing *et al.*, 2003; Slade, 2002, 2006), for instance, is a preventive group intervention programme for parents of infants, toddlers and preschoolers. The programme aims to support the parents and enhance the parent–infant relationship by promoting parental capacities for reflective functioning. The Minding the Baby programme (Slade, 2002, 2006; Slade *et al.*, 2005b; Sadler *et al.*, 2006), in turn, is an interdisciplinary, relationship-based home visiting programme using a mentalization-based approach to promote the reflective capacities of young mothers at risk.

Partly inspired by these programmes, MBT-P specifically aims at improving PRF in parents with BPD. As noted, a fundamental assumption of the mentalization-based approach to BPD is that the attachment system of patients with BPD is readily – and often too readily – triggered, resulting in a deactivation of controlled mentalizing. This feature might explain the fast attachment of many BPD patients to others, often followed by subsequent disillusion, anger and resentment. Importantly, the challenges inherent in the parent–infant relationship are likely to be a main trigger of the attachment system in parents with BPD, which may in turn compromise their mentalizing capacities. It is therefore our fundamental belief that promoting a mentalizing stance in parents with BPD can enhance their abilities to envision the mind of their children, helping them create a better understanding of their children, which is likely to improve the parent–child relationship and ultimately foster child development. Based on studies reviewed above, one can moreover expect that enhancing PRF will not only have a beneficial effect on the parent–child relationship, but may also have a preventive effect with regard to possible maladaptive development of the child.

Mentalization-based treatment for parents (MBT-P)

Inspired by the Parents First and Minding the Baby programmes, we developed a parent–infant module that can be flexibly added to MBT-IOP. MBT-P combines both a curative focus with regard to borderline features in the parent, as well as a preventive focus with regard to the parent–infant relationship and the child's development. Moreover, as some children of BPD parents may suffer from various emotional and behavioural problems, in some cases MBT-P may also have a curative focus with regard to the child.

The target population for MBT-P consists of parents seeking treatment for their BPD. We use the term 'parents' in this context to refer to the primary attachment figure of the child, i.e. the biological, adoptive or foster parent. Moreover, the programme is aimed at both mothers and fathers. MBT-P was primarily developed for parents and their infants or children aged zero to four. The focus is on the parent and his or her ability for parental mentalization and not directly on the child itself. If the child has a medical condition or psychological problems that need specific attention or extra care, the child is typically referred to specialized care (e.g. a paediatrician or child psychotherapist). In this case, however, we consider it extremely important to discuss and reach consensus on a common approach. Simply combining child therapy, for instance, and MBT-P without a coherent strategy shared by all professionals involved in the complex treatment of parent and child may lead to confusion in the parent, the child or children, and professionals.

Because of its focus on the parent, MBT-P can be started during pregnancy, at birth, or after arrival of the child. We consider it highly preferable to establish a working alliance with the parent before childbirth (in the case of biological parenthood) or child arrival (in the case of adoptive and foster parenthood), because MBT-P's focus on the parent–infant relationship is often experienced as very threatening. This seems especially true for parents with BPD, as they often fear that their parental capacities will be criticized or condemned by therapists or child protective services, often reinforcing their fear of child placement. Although these fears prevent parents from seeking appropriate professional help for parenting problems, they are not entirely irrational as many of these patients are under the supervision of child protective services and/or live with the constant threat that their child will be removed from their care. Thus, establishing a therapeutic alliance with the parent as early as possible provides the therapist with more time and thus opportunities to help engage the parent in the treatment process. Moreover, this additionally helps the therapist to develop a more sophisticated model of the patient's mind, including his or her fears, resistances and other transference tracers possibly leading to commitment problems or destructive behaviour. This has often proved extremely helpful in repairing possible ruptures in the therapeutic alliance and in sustaining continued motivation after childbirth or arrival, when arousal levels are typically much higher, and parents are more inclined to refuse help or drop out of treatment prematurely.

Structure of mentalization-based treatment for parents

Ingredients

MBT-P is a reflective parenting programme combining MBT-IOP and a parent–infant module. The structure and principles of MBT-IOP are described in detail elsewhere (Bateman & Fonagy, 2006). Below, we will only summarize some aspects of MBT-IOP that are relevant to understand the structure of MBT-P.

MBT-IOP consists of group psychotherapy and individual psychotherapy sessions. If necessary, pharmacotherapy is integrated in the therapy. The twice-weekly group sessions last for one hour, and the weekly individual sessions have a duration of 45 minutes. Both individual and group sessions have a clear and consistent focus on enhancing the patient's mentalizing capacity. Although this often entails a focus on mentalizing with regard to specific relationships, parental mentalization is typically not an explicit focus of MBT-IOP.

The parent–infant module specifically focuses on PRF by using video-feedback and other mentalization promoting techniques, and includes 45 minutes of individual parent–infant psychotherapy once every two weeks and a group training of six 90-minutes sessions scheduled over a two-month time span. During the entire treatment period, home visits, telephone calls, and other outreach activities are used as an agreed part of the treatment plan, for example, as part of the engagement process, or to repair or enhance the therapeutic alliance. These activities are generally performed by a psychosocial nurse.

In Viersprong, there are three MBT-IOP groups of nine patients each. Each MBT-IOP group is allowed to include a maximum of three caregivers who have the parent–infant module integrated in their treatment programme. We have deliberately chosen to include patients with and without the parent–infant module in standard MBT-IOP, as the focus in standard MBT should be on BPD difficulties and not on parenting. If a standard MBT-IOP group consisted only of caregivers receiving the parent–infant module, the focus would inevitably shift toward parenting, with the risk of not addressing their individual BPD-related needs.

The parent–infant module and the standard MBT-IOP are offered by different therapists. By working with different therapists, the differentiation of the foci on individual and parent–infant themes respectively is ensured. An additional, more practical reason is that parent–infant therapists are child psychotherapists specialized in the treatment of parent–child relationships, but also preferably have experience in the treatment of adult BPD, whereas the MBT-IOP therapists need to be specialized in the treatment of adult BPD only. Both have received extensive training in MBT.

In our setting, an MBT-P team typically consists of three MBT therapists (i.e. two for MBT-IOP and one for the parent–infant module), a psychosocial nurse, a psychiatrist and a supervisor (who enhances adherence to the mentalizing model and the reflective stance within the staff). It is important that the various therapists who are involved in the treatment of individual patients closely collaborate, so as to ensure the coherence and consistency of the treatment. Coherence and consistency are essential: (a) to prevent splitting between therapists; (b) for the effective integration of the various therapy components; and (c) to prevent confusion in the professionals involved with regard to responsibilities and focus. Confusion and inconsistencies between therapists may create intense distress in the BPD patients, leading to destabilization and possibly crises.

Treatment planning

At the beginning of treatment, the individual psychotherapist and patient collaboratively formulate a treatment plan. This consists of five individualized treatment goals with respect to the following themes: (a) engagement in therapy; (b) psychiatric complaints; (c) relational difficulties; (d) self-destructive behaviour; (e) frequent hospitalizations and other health care consumption. The treatment goals are primarily described in terms of mental states underlying behaviour. During the individual parent–infant psychotherapy, this treatment plan will be complemented with treatment themes regarding parenthood and the parent–infant relationship with respect to both parental strengths as well as parental vulnerabilities.

Every four weeks, the treatment plan is discussed with the entire staff, and treatment plan evaluations with the entire staff and the patient are held every three months. Such evaluations are 'moments of attunement' between patient and staff, in order: (a) to systematically evaluate treatment goals and progress; (b) to revise treatment goals if necessary; (c) to reflect on patient and therapist experiences in treatment; (d) to discuss whether the therapy still meets the patient's needs, and – if not – how to change it. When the child receives treatment outside of the MBT setting, the child therapist is invited for the treatment plan evaluation, again to ensure coherence and consistency of the treatment.

In addition to the treatment plan, the patient develops with the help of a psychosocial nurse a crisis plan from a mentalizing perspective, in which the infant receives a central place (i.e. 'What do I have to do with my baby when I am in crisis or emotionally upset?').

Individual parent–infant psychotherapy

During the individual parent–infant module therapy sessions, the parent is asked to bring the infant or child to the therapy. In these sessions there is a continuous focus on mentalizing about self (as parent), child and the parent–infant relationship. The parent–infant module can be divided into three treatment phases: the initial phase, the middle phase and the final phase.

In the initial phase, the overall aim is assessment of PRF and engaging the patient in treatment. Specific processes in this phase include: building a working alliance, psycho-education about mentalization and the MBT-P treatment programme, and establishing therapeutic goals with regard to the parent–infant relationship.

In the middle phase, the primary aim is enhancing PRF, with interventions focusing on the parent–child relationship. During this phase, the therapist's main interventions are based on video-feedback to promote PRF. Video-feedback is a therapeutic intervention which has become increasingly common over the past years in the field of parent–infant therapy (for a review, see Svanberg, 2009). In the Minding the Baby programme, for instance, video-feedback is used to increase PRF, and has shown encouraging results in terms of improvements in mothers' sensitive responsiveness (Slade *et al.*, 2005c). Video-feedback may be particularly effective in promoting mentalization, as it forces parents to focus on their internal mental states and that of their child from a third-person perspective (Luyten *et al.*, 2009).

Video-feedback interventions in the parent–infant psychotherapy are based on free-play interactions. Moreover, the patient is given a video camera to tape 'difficult' moments at home with which he or she struggles (e.g. eating or sleeping time), or moments in which parental strengths are reflected. Subsequently, therapist and patient watch the video tapes together and reflect on specific moments, attending to both parental strengths and vulnerabilities as well as child characteristics, and their interplay. The focus, as noted, is always on the mental state of the parent and child, and particularly on reflecting together, in a collaborative way, about what is happening in the parent–child interaction in the actual moment.

In the final phase of treatment, the patient and individual therapist collaboratively develop a follow-up plan aiming to consolidate and further enhance PRF, and to further stimulate parental responsibility and independent parental functioning. The follow-up plan should focus on accomplishments as well as aspects of parental functioning that deserve further attention.

Explicit mentalizing group training

In addition to the individual psychotherapy, the parent–infant module includes an additional explicit mentalizing group training consisting of six group sessions. The course aims to address the following themes:

- *BPD and mentalization* (i.e. what BPD means for the patient and others; what is mentalizing; how mentalizing abilities may be lost and restored; how BPD and failures in mentalization can affect the relationship with the child).
- *Parenthood* (i.e. what is it like to be a parent; struggles and strengths in parenthood; difficult moments during parenthood, for example, how to deal with a crying baby; how to find out what your infant is trying to communicate).
- *Interplay of thoughts, feelings and intentions* (i.e. acknowledgement of the fact that even very young children have their own thoughts, feelings and intentions; the relationship between these thoughts, feelings and intentions on the one hand and behaviours on the other; intersection of minds; the fact that parent and child have separate minds, and can disagree or have different ideas about the same thing).
- *Attachment and intergenerational transmission* (i.e. what is attachment and how does it feel; the transformation of being a child into being a parent; how your own childhood can affect parenthood; ghosts and angels in the nursery).
- *Separation–individuation* (i.e. how to deal with/interpret moments of separation and individuation; how to recognize these moments).
- *Emotional development and regulation* (i.e. parenthood can provoke strong emotions; how to recognize these emotions and how to deal with them; the developmental path of children).

Every workshop session starts with an introduction of the themes mentioned above. This psycho-educational component is not a one-way ‘telling’ the patient what he or she needs to know, but stimulates the participants' mentalization in a structured manner about the themes. Exercises are arranged using personal experiences whenever possible. The focus remains on enhancing the patient's reflecting thinking about their own or others' experiences, supporting each other, and on highlighting and creating alternative perspectives.

Therapeutic stance and intervention principles in MBT-P

This section describes the therapeutic stance and intervention principles used to promote parental mentalizing. As noted, these descriptions are based on (1) existing mentalization-based interventions for parents and their infants (Goyette-Ewing *et al.*, 2003; Sadler *et al.*, 2006; Slade, 2006; Slade *et al.*, 2005b, 2005c); (2) intervention principles for MBT as described by Bateman and Fonagy (2004, 2006); (3) our own clinical experience in working with these patients.

Therapeutic stance

The essence of the therapeutic stance in MBT is adopting a 'not knowing' stance (Bateman & Fonagy, 2010). This means that the therapist should explicitly and actively identify, legitimize and accept different or alternative perspectives together with the patient about what is happening in the moment. In doing so, the therapist asks for detailed descriptions of experience (i.e. 'What is that feeling like?'), rather than explanations (i.e. 'Why do you think that?'). Lack of clarity in what the patient is describing must be addressed. Further, it is important that the therapist monitors his or her own mentalizing failures, as such failures are likely to happen in the face of a non-mentalizing patient and parent. Consequently, occasional enactments by the therapist are acceptable concomitants of the therapeutic alliance. In case of mentalization breakdowns, the therapist and patient should 'stop and rewind', and explore the incident.

During the parent–infant therapy, the therapist has three relationships to account for, namely the relationship between therapist and parent, between therapist and infant or child, and between parent and infant or child. The overall aim is to enhance PRF by enhancing the parent's capacity to mentalize about self, other (child, therapist) and the parent–infant interaction.

The therapist attempts to help the patient to realize that mental states are opaque by modelling a not knowing stance, tolerating uncertainty, and also stimulating curiosity and motivation to seek out mental states. The therapist attempts to evoke curiosity in the parent about the infant's experiences, and to help him or her recognize that these experiences are separate from their own. The following example illustrates this stance, with special attention to the three relationships that are always involved in working with the patient and his or her child.

During one session, a mother explains that she has difficulties managing her anger when she is feeding her five-month-old baby girl: 'Before I start feeding her I intend to stay calm, but when she spits out the pacifier for the thousandth time, I really lose it. And then she smiles at me like she is trying to say: "Haha, got you there, didn't I?"' The therapist tries to evoke curiosity about the infant's experience by asking the mother why her daughter would do this. At first she answers: 'I don't know, I think she is just trying to bully me. She just wants attention and that's why she is trying to prolong the feeding process.' The therapist then responds: 'Oh, do you really think that? That's awful if you feel it that way. I don't know, but could there be other reasons why she might spit out her pacifier?' The mother answers: 'I don't know, I think she just wants attention. These feeding moments are often the only moments during the day in which we really have contact. We don't have a lot of contact. I don't really know how to act when I'm with her, she's just a baby and can't talk, how would I know what she wants or likes? . . . Hey, maybe that's it, maybe she is just trying to make contact with me, maybe she misses contact and grasps this opportunity to play with me?' In this example, it is clear how this mother's emerging curiosity about her child's mental states led to an alternative perspective, a better understanding of the child and a transformation of the parental representations of the infant.

The pedagogical stance is another important aspect of the therapeutic stance. Pedagogical interactions on the part of the parent can be seen as implicit teachings regarding the infant's mind, in particular with regard to emotional states. For instance, the child learns about his mental states or emotions (e.g. sadness) by observing his or her parental reactions to these affects (e.g. containment and marked affect mirroring). Ostensive cues, such as eye contact, 'motherese' and marked affect mirroring, directly foster the infant's interpersonal learning, which leads to mentalized representations of his or her emotional states (Allen *et al.*, 2008). The capacity for the parent to use ostensive communication and take the pedagogical stance entails PRF, which makes pedagogical learning an important aspect of the parent–infant therapy.

During the sessions, the therapist therefore should adopt the pedagogical stance and use ostensive communication as a model for the parent (i.e. by marked affect mirroring towards the infant). It is important to note that the pedagogical stance is different from providing pedagogic advice or developmental knowledge, which is avoided in MBT-P. Advising or instructing the patient what he or she needs to know and do is not compatible with the mentalizing therapeutic stance and is not considered to be likely to enhance mentalizing. For instance, in the sixth session of the explicit mentalizing group training the therapist provides some psycho-education about the development of children. In doing so, the main focus is to encourage the parent to think and wonder about the development of his own child in order to create an understanding of the child, the child's development, and the interaction between them.

Focus on current mental states

Interventions should be simple and easy to understand, actively engaging the patient and keeping in mind the patient's deficits in mentalizing capacity. The interventions are focused on mental states rather than on behaviour, and are related to current activities or interpersonal/parental interactions. The primary aim of treatment is to help the parent give meaning to the infant's behaviour, to understand her or his child in terms of what she or he is feeling and thinking, and not in terms of how she or he is acting. Together with the parent, the therapist should observe the infant's signals, and try to reflect on what the infant is communicating and how this affects the parent. This entails that during the therapy session the therapist and patient continuously switch between mentalizing about self, other (infant or child) and the parent–infant interaction, illustrated in the following example.

A 39-year-old father complains about his 3-year-old son's behaviour during a parent–infant therapy session. The little boy is pulling all the napkins out of the napkin box and throwing them in the garbage can. The father gets angry and demands his son to stop. To the therapist he says: 'Why doesn't he behave like a good boy? He's always bullying me with his bad behaviour!' In this example, the father is clearly talking about his son in terms of behaviour, and not wondering about the underlying mental states. It is important to try to shift this behavioural focus to a focus on the underlying mental states. In this example, the therapist has to help the parent reflect on what is happening in the actual moment. First, the therapist can focus on the mental state of the parent: How does he feel at this moment and what makes him feel that way? Next, the therapist can ask the father to reflect on the mental state of his son: What makes the child behave like this? Is he really bullying his father or can we think of other reasons? The therapist can help the parent to find alternative explanations by modelling reflectiveness (see below) and engaging the child in this process (e.g. by saying: 'Oh, it seems that you have found a funny new little game.').

Focus on affect

In MBT, the focus on affects means attempting to grasp the affect in the immediacy of the moment, not so much in its relation to what the parent is saying (content of story), but primarily as it relates to what is happening now, in the session between parent and child. Identifying the current feeling helps bridge the gap between the primary affective experience and its symbolic representation, strengthening the secondary representational system of the parent, and indirectly of the child. In exploring the affects within a concrete situation in the session, the therapist keeps his mentalizing stance, asking questions such as: 'What happened, what do you make of that?' 'How does that leave you feeling now?' 'What do you think your child is feeling? Or felt?' and 'How do you know that?'

Exploring concrete situations can provoke strong feelings within the parent. Experiencing these current emotions, labelling, differentiating and representing them, and placing them within a present context are important keys to change. During this process the therapist must remain flexible, keeping possible failures of mentalizing of the parent in mind, and adjusting the complexity and emotional intensity of interventions according to the intensity of the patient's emotional arousal. Too much arousal leaves the parent vulnerable to deactivation of controlled mentalizing. Hence, it will be more helpful to explore a situation in the (recent) past and to provide adequate supportive and empathic interventions, lowering the arousal and reinstating mentalizing. During the video-feedback sessions, arousal levels are typically very high as, for instance, many parents fear the judgement of the therapist. While watching some video fragments, the parent's emotional arousal can be reduced by supportive techniques such as praise and empathy, and by switching between past affects and thoughts (e.g. 'What did you feel, when you ignored your daughter?') and current affects and thoughts (e.g. 'What do you feel now, while watching this fragment?').

Modelling parental reflectiveness

In MBT-P, it is important to model reflective functioning by representing the child's mental states to the caregiver. This can be done by focusing on the infant's internal states and intentions. The following excerpt from the treatment of a 25-year-old mother with BPD and her six-month-old son illustrates this principle.

In the first session, the mother, her baby, and the therapist are sitting on the floor, discussing the mother's feelings about the MBT-P programme. The mother expresses difficulties in trusting the therapist and in understanding how the treatment programme could help her with her own problems and those in the relationship with her son. She talks about her many fears, which all seem to be related to the theme of abandonment. She has a lack of self-esteem and fears that her son will reject her for not being a good mother. She also fears that something bad might happen to him, or that someone (for instance, the therapist) would take her boy away from her. While talking to the therapist, she fearfully holds her son in front of her with his face away from the therapist, avoiding any contact between the therapist and her baby. Her son keeps turning and facing the therapist and then smiles at her. The mother seems to feel very threatened by this. She repeatedly turns his head back to her and tries to make contact with him, however unsuccessfully so because the boy keeps turning his head back again towards the therapist.

The tension in the room increases dramatically; feelings of anger, fear, sadness and helplessness confuse the mother. At this moment, the therapist attempts to articulate the infant's internal experience to the mother in a non-threatening way by speaking on behalf of the baby: 'But mommy, I want to see what you see. . . Who is that lady? I don't know her, let's take a look at her. . .'. The mother smiles a little awkwardly. Then the therapist says to the infant, using her normal voice: 'Isn't all of this exciting, a new playroom, a new face. You want to look around and explore all these new things, don't you? I understand that.' These interventions quickly lower the tension and allow the mother to explore her feelings of being threatened, as well as her lack of trust, and her fears of loss and abandonment.

Focus on parental strengths

MBT-P focuses as much as possible on the parent's strengths. Highlighting parental strengths is seen as a reassuring and supportive intervention, helping to lower arousal levels and create possibilities to further enhance mentalization. The parent will more easily accept and learn from interventions when feeling reinforced rather than criticized. For example, the therapist might compliment and reinforce the parent when he or she offers adequate comfort and containment to a distressed or crying child.

Positive reinforcing also creates opportunities to focus on parental vulnerabilities. In the example above, the distress in the child was caused by the parent's behaviour prior to the crying. After the reassurance, the therapist can focus on this interaction by rewinding the session to the moment before the child started crying (stop, rewind and explore) and retracing the interaction, focusing on stimulating reflection of mental states of the child, parent and their interaction.

Challenge and praise

Finally, when the therapist observes 'pseudo-mentalizing' in the parent (i.e. when the parent considers mental states, but with no connection to actual reality), it is important to recognize and challenge the patient, thereby reinstating mentalizing. For example, a BPD mother with a four-year-old daughter explains her daughter's problem behaviour in terms of general causes she has picked up from reading magazines and watching television programmes. In doing so, she seems to have no notion of her daughter's mind. Such attributions should be identified, helping parents to take a more mentalizing stance.

At moments of positive mentalizing on the part of the parent, it can be very helpful and motivating to reinforce mentalizing and to help explore its beneficial effects on the parent, child and the relationship. For instance, after viewing a patient struggling to understand, and reflect on, the mental states of her upset son, the therapist responds with, 'Wow, you really seem to understand him [the child], even now when he's really upset. How does this make you feel? How is this helping you? Is this changing the way you feel about his anger?' Doing this enables the parent to experience how a better understanding will help in managing strong affects and altering negative representations.

Mentalizing in the current/here-and-now parent–infant relationship

An important rule in working with parents is to first let the interaction unfold, allowing the parent to take the lead, which at the same time reveals the particular parent–child relationship. The therapist should resist intervening immediately, for example, when a lack of parental sensitivity is clear from the start or if the parent displays behaviours that disrupt the child. At times this can be very difficult, but it should be kept in mind that immediate interventions will not be helpful in the long run. What happens in the therapy room is also likely to happen at home, highlighting the importance of taking such an interaction very seriously and viewing these disruptive moments in the session as starting points for reflective thinking about the parent–infant relationship. Focusing on these situations in the room at the moment, the therapist can encourage the parent to think about the relationship they are in at the current moment (with their child) with the aim to focus their attention on another mind, the mind of their child, and to help them reflect on their own perception of themselves, their child and their relationship, and contrast these perceptions with other possible alternative perspectives.

Conclusion

MBT-P is a relatively new treatment programme targeted at parents with BPD who primarily seek treatment for their own problems and complaints. Although MBT-P includes infants and children aged zero to four in the treatment, the focus is on parental mentalization and not directly on the child itself. This chapter described the theoretical background and development of the programme, as well as the structure and intervention principles. Currently, we are piloting the programme, developing a manual, and planning a study aimed at evaluating its (cost-) effectiveness. In this study, we will compare developmental pathways and outcomes of children of parents receiving MBT-P versus children of parents receiving standard

MBT alone. Based on our first experiences with MBT-P, the treatment programme seems promising, but further research is definitely needed to substantiate these impressions.

References

Allen, J. G., Fonagy, P., & Bateman, A. W. (2008). *Mentalizing in clinical practice*. Arlington VA: American Psychiatric Publishing.

Arnott, B., & Meins, E. (2007). Links among antenatal attachment representations, postnatal mind-mindedness, and infant attachment security: A preliminary study of mothers and fathers. *Bulletin of the Menninger Clinic*, 71(2), 132–149.

Bales, D., Smits, M., Verheul, R., van Busschbach, J. J., van Beek, N., Willemsen, S., *et al.* (in press). Treatment outcome of 18-month, day hospital mentalization-based treatment (MBT) in patients with severe borderline personality disorder in the Netherlands. *Journal of Personality Disorders.*

Bateman, A. W., & Fonagy, P. (1999). The effectiveness of partial hospitalization in the treatment of borderline personality disorder – a randomised controlled trial. *American Journal of Psychiatry*, 156, 1563–1569.

Bateman, A. W., & Fonagy, P. (2001). Treatment of borderline personality disorder with psychoanalytically oriented partial hospitalization: An 18-month follow-up. *American Journal of Psychiatry*, 158(1), 36–42.

Bateman, A. W., & Fonagy, P. (2004). *Psychotherapy for borderline personality disorder: Mentalization-based treatment*. Oxford: Oxford University Press.

Bateman, A. W., & Fonagy, P. (2006). *Mentalization-based treatment for borderline personality disorder: A practical guide*. Oxford: Oxford University Press.

Bateman, A. W., & Fonagy, P. (2008). 8-year follow-up of patients treated for borderline personality disorder: Mentalization-based treatment versus treatment as usual. *American Journal of Psychiatry*, 165(5), 631–638.

Bateman, A. W., & Fonagy, P. (2009). Randomized controlled trial of outpatient mentalization-based treatment versus structured clinical management for borderline personality disorder. *American Journal of Psychiatry*, 166(12), 1355–1364.

Bateman, A. W., & Fonagy, P. (2010). Mentalization-based treatment for borderline personality disorder. *World Psychiatry*, 9(1), 11–15.

Black, D. W., Blum, N., Pfohl, B., & Hale, N. (2004). Suicidal behaviour in borderline personality disorder: Prevalence, risk factors, prediction, and prevention. *Journal of Personality Disorders*, 18(3), 226–239.

Ensink, K., & Mayes, L. C. (2010). The development of mentalisation in children from a theory of mind perspective. *Psychoanalytic Inquiry*, 30, 301–337.

Fonagy, P., & Luyten, P. (2009) A developmental, mentalization-based approach to the understanding and treatment of borderline personality disorder. *Development and Psychopathology*, 21(4), 1355–1381.

Fonagy, P., & Target, M. (2005). Bridging the transmission gap: An end to an important mystery of attachment research? *Attachment & Human Development*, 7(3), 333–343.

Fonagy, P., Luyten, P., Bateman, A., Gergely, G., Strathearn, L., Target, M., *et al.* (2010). Attachment and personality pathology. In J. F. Clarkin, P. Fonagy &

G. O. Gabbard (Eds.), *Psychodynamic psychotherapy for personality disorders. A clinical handbook* (pp. 37–87). Washington, DC: American Psychiatric Publishing.

Fonagy, P., Luyten, P., & Strathearn, L. (2011). Mentalization and the roots of borderline personality disorder in infancy. In H. E. Fitzgerald, K. Puura, M. Tomlinson, & C. Paul (Eds.), *International perspectives on children and mental health: Volume 1: Development and context* (pp. 129–154). New York: Praeger.

Gottman, J. M., Katz, L. F., & Hooven, D. (1996). Parental meta-emotion philosophy and the emotional life of families: Theoretical models and preliminary data. *Journal of Family Psychology*, 10, 243–268.

Goyette-Ewing, M., Slade, A., Knoebber, K., Gilliam, W., Truman, S., & Mayes, L. (2003), Parents first: A developmental parenting program. Unpublished manuscript. New Haven, CT: Yale Child Study Centre.

Grienenberger, J., Kelly, K., & Slade, A. (2005). Maternal reflective functioning, mother–infant affective communication, and infant attachment: Exploring the link between mental states and observed caregiving behavior in the intergenerational transmission of attachment. *Attachment and Human Development*, 7(3), 299–311.

Grootens, K. P., van Luijtelaar, G., Buitelaar, J. K., van der Laan, A., Hummelen, J. W., & Verkes, R. J. (2008). Inhibition errors in borderline personality disorder with psychotic-like symptoms. *Progress in Neuro-Psychopharmacology and Biological Psychiatry*, 32(1), 267–273.

Hill, J., Pilkonis, P., Morse, J., Feske, U., Reynolds, S., Hope, H., *et al.* (2008). Social domain dysfunction and disorganization in borderline personality disorder. *Psychological Medicine*, 38(1), 135–146.

Katz, L. F., & Windecker-Nelson, B. (2004). Parental meta-emotion philosophy in families with conduct-problem children. *Journal of Abnormal Child Psychology*, 32, 385–398.

Levy, K. N., Beeney, J. E., & Temes, C. M. (2011). Attachment and its vicissitudes in borderline personality disorder. *Current Psychiatry Reports*, 13, 50–59.

Linehan, M. M. (1993). *Cognitive-behavioural treatment of borderline personality disorder*. New York: Guilford Press.

Luyten, P., Fonagy, P., Vermote, R., & Lowyck, B. (2009). The assessment of mentalization. In P. Fonagy & A. Bateman (Eds.), *Mentalizing in mental health practice* (pp. 43–66). Washington, DC: American Psychiatric Press.

Macfie, J. (2009). Development in children and adolescents whose mothers have borderline personality disorder. *Child Development Perspectives*, 3(1), 66–71.

Meins, E. (1997). *Security of attachment and the social development of cognition*. Hove, UK: Psychology Press.

Meins, E. (1999). Sensitivity, security and internal working models: Bridging the transmission gap. *Attachment and Human Development*, 1, 325–342.

Meins, E., Fernyhough, C., Fradley, E., & Tuckey, M. (2001). Rethinking maternal sensitivity: Mother's comments on infant's mental processes predict security of attachment at 12 months. *Journal of Child Psychology and Psychiatry*, 42, 637–648.

Meins, E., Fernyhough, C., Wainwright, R., Das Gupta, M., Fradley, E., & Tuckey, M. (2002). Maternal mind-mindedness and attachment security as predictors of theory of mind understanding. *Child Development*, 73, 1715–1726.

Meins, E., Fernyhough, C., Wainwright, R., Clark-Carter, D., Das Gupta, M., Fradley, E., *et al.* (2003). Pathways to understanding mind: Construct validity and predictive validity of maternal mind-mindedness. *Child Development*, 74, 1194–1211.

Reisch, T., Ebner-Priemer, U. W., Tschacher, W., Bohus, M., & Linehan, M. M. (2008). Sequences of emotions in patients with borderline personality disorder. *Acta Psychiatrica Scandinavica*, 118(1), 42–48.

Rosenblum, K. L., McDonough, S. C., Sameroff, A. J., & Muzik, M. (2008). Reflection in thought and action: Maternal parenting reflectivity predicts mind-minded comments and interactive behavior. *Infant Mental Health Journal*, 29(4), 362–376.

Sadler, L. S., Slade, A., & Mayes, L. C. (2006). Minding the baby: A mentalization-based parenting program. In J. G. Allen & P. Fonagy (Eds.), *Handbook of mentalization-based treatment* (pp. 271–288). Chichester: Wiley.

Sharp, C., & Fonagy, P. (2008). The parent's capacity to treat the child as a psychological agent: Constructs, measures and implications for developmental psychopathology. *Social Development*, 17(3), 737–754.

Sharp, C., Fonagy, P., & Goodyer, I. M. (2006). Imagining your child's mind: Psychosocial adjustment and mothers' ability to predict their children's attributional response styles. *British Journal of Developmental Psychology*, 24, 197–214.

Slade, A. (2002). Keeping the baby in mind: A critical factor in perinatal mental health. In A. Slade, L. Mayes & N. Epperson (Eds.), special issue on perinatal mental health. *Zero to Three*, 10–16.

Slade, A. (2005). Parental reflective functioning: An introduction. *Attachment and Human Development*, 7(3), 269–281.

Slade, A. (2006). Reflective parenting programs: Theory and development. *Psychoanalytic Inquiry*, 26(4), 640–657.

Slade, A., Grienenberger, J., Bernbach, E., Levy, D., & Locker, A. (2005a). Maternal reflective functioning, attachment, and the transmission gap: A preliminary study. *Attachment and Human Development*, 7(3), 283–298.

Slade, A., Sadler, L., De Dios-Kenn, C., Webb, D., Currier-Ezepchick, J., & Mayes, L. (2005b). Minding the baby: A reflective parenting program. *Psychoanalytic Study of the Child*, 60, 74–100.

Slade, A., Sadler, L., & Mayes, L. (2005c). Minding the baby: Enhancing parental reflective functioning in a nursing/mental health home visiting program. In L. Berlin, Y. Zin, L. Amya-Jackson & M. T. Greenberg (Eds.), *Enhancing early attachments: Theory, research, intervention and policy* (pp. 152–177). London: Guilford Press.

Steele, H., & Siever, L. (2010). An attachment perspective on borderline personality disorder: Advances in gene-environment considerations. *Current Psychiatry Reports*, 12, 61–67.

Suchman, N., DeCoste, C., Castiglioni, N., Legow, N., & Mayes, L. (2008). The Mothers and Toddlers Program: Preliminary findings from an attachment-based parenting intervention for substance-abusing mothers. *Psychoanalytic Psychology*, 25, 499–517.

Suchman, N. E., DeCoste, C., Castiglioni, N., McMahon, T. J., Rounsaville, B., & Mayes, L. (2010). The Mothers and Toddlers Program, an attachment-based parenting intervention for substance using women: Post-treatment results from a randomized clinical pilot. *Attachment and Human Development*, 12(5), 483–504.

Svanberg, P. O. (2009). Promoting a secure attachment through early screening and interventions: A partnership approach. In J. Barlow & P. O. Svanberg (Eds.), *Baby in mind. Infant mental health in practice* (pp. 185–198). London: Routledge.

Chapter 5

Minding the family mind

The development and initial evaluation of mentalization-based treatment for families

Emma Keaveny, Nick Midgley, Eia Asen, Dickon Bevington, Pasco Fearon, Peter Fonagy, Ruth Jennings-Hobbs and Sally Wood

> Maybe you can remember an afternoon from your childhood where you created a whole world in your bedroom? Perhaps it was a battle between the soldiers and your collection of farm animals? The duvet hanging over the side of the bed has become a cliff and a yellow beach towel is the desert with your mother's blue scarf as a river. The soldiers are lined up at the top of the cliff and the animals, marshalled by your favourite teddy bear, make their way across the river in saucers.

As children, most of us have a great capacity to operate in what Fonagy and Target (1996) have described as 'pretend mode'. Of course we know that the duvet isn't really a cliff; and if it is time for tea, we can take the saucers back to the kitchen without really believing that the toy animals are going to drown without their boats. But whilst we are playing, the reality of the game is all that matters – and being able to 'play with reality' in such a way is a vital part of growing up.

Expanding one's capacity to 'play with reality' – and entering into the world of others to see things from their perspectives – is an important stage in psychosocial development and is an enormously valuable part of adult life too. Research has shown us that an individual's ability to do this can be significantly impaired by trauma, abuse and stress (Luyten *et al.*, 2009). Many of the families who are referred to child and adolescent mental health services may have lost this capacity to 'play' with different perspectives. Even when this has not been part of the cause of the difficulties that they are presenting it is most often a contributing factor in the maintenance of the problem. As such, regaining such a capacity may be a vital aspect of helping families to overcome their difficulties.

This chapter will describe the development and initial evaluation of an approach to working with families which is adapted from mentalization-based treatment (MBT; Bateman & Fonagy, 2004), a model of treatment originally developed in the context of work with adults with borderline personality disorder (BPD). Mentalization-based treatment for families

(MBT-F)[1] has been developed as a brief intervention devised by the Anna Freud Centre, the Marlborough Family Service in London and Baylor Medical College in the USA. We will begin by offering some description of the service as it has developed at the Anna Freud Centre, before going on to describe some of the key components of the model, including: the importance of the therapist's 'mentalizing stance'; how we aim to 'hold the balance'; and the use of the 'mentalizing loop'. The chapter will end by briefly outlining some key findings from the initial evaluation of the service, and will include some of the lessons we have drawn from our work with families so far.

Introduction to the Family Support Service

As a charity in the UK dedicated to caring for young minds, the Anna Freud Centre is not only a centre for research and training, but also runs a number of clinical services in which new approaches to working with children and families can be developed and routinely evaluated. For families of school-aged children, the first port of call for concerned parents or carers is our telephone-based parent consultation service, which was set up in 2009 to offer free, easily accessed and expert advice to families in distress in the local area. Feedback from parents indicated that for a significant proportion of these families the 30-minute telephone consultation, which is followed up by a letter summarizing the key points discussed during the call, seemed to be enough to get things 'back on track', and no further intervention was needed. Parents have commented especially on the importance of being listened to non-judgementally and having an opportunity to think about their family's situation from a different perspective. For some of the parents who contact our consultation service, however, it is clear that the problems are significant or longstanding, and that further help is needed beyond the initial consultation, which may include a referral to our MBT-F service.

Mentalization-based treatment for families (MBT-F)

MBT-F is an approach to clinical work which aims at increasing the mentalizing capacity of families, supporting them to clarify the specific thoughts,

1 In previous publications MBT-F has been known as SMART (short-term mentalizing and relational therapy; see Fearon *et al.*, 2006) or mentalization-based family therapy (MBFT). In order to make it clear how this approach relates to the 'family' of mentalization-based treatments, and to clarify that a short course in this approach is not equivalent to a full family therapy training, the approach has been renamed mentalization-based treatment – family (MBT-F). At the Anna Freud Centre, the work of the MBT-F team is generously funded by the John Lyon's Charity and the Priory Foundation.

feelings, wishes and beliefs that underpin the habitual attitudes and behaviours which may be contributing to the difficulties they are experiencing.

When it was first developed, one of the aims of MBT-F was to offer a short-term (6–10 session) model of work that would be appropriate for a wide range of children and families. We keep to a minimum the number of formal exclusion criteria, but make it clear to all families from the beginning that our focus will be on family relationships, and working on improving these in order to support them to understand and manage the specific difficulties or symptoms their children may be presenting. We get many referrals, for example, from families who have recently gone through a divorce or separation and where a parent is concerned about a sudden change in their child's behaviour such as an increase in verbal and physical aggression.

As well as being an adaptation of MBT, the work integrates aspects of systemic, cognitive and psychodynamic therapies with the latest research on the capacity to mentalize in both parents and children. Clinicians familiar with cognitive behavioural therapy will recognize much of the emphasis on making links between cognitions and behaviour; whilst those from a psychodynamic background will certainly be aware of the importance of working with the 'here and now' (Sandler, 1976) and the dynamics in the consulting room. Given that this is a family-based intervention, there is a particular debt to the various traditions within family therapy. Those working from a systemic perspective will see many techniques familiar to them, from 'joining' (Minuchin, 1974), to focusing on exceptions to symptomatic behaviours (de Shazer, 1982), and including the importance of 'curiosity' (Cecchin, 1987), and 'circular questioning' (Selvini Palazzoli *et al.*, 1980). Furthermore, an increased focus on working with emotions in the 'here and now' is gaining pace though it is not usually a priority and is often linked with psychoanalytic practices (Pocock, 2009; Rober, 1999). There are also systemic practitioners who have explored the therapeutic territory which transcends the seemingly clear distinctions between systemic, psychoanalytic and cognitive approaches and helpfully explored common ground (for example, Donovan, 2009; Larner, 2000).

Despite these debts to other models, we do believe that MBT-F has some distinctive features which are different from but complementary to these other approaches. The emphasis on mentalization can enhance the effectiveness of family-based treatments by providing a way to get around common blocks in therapy and making family members more receptive to tuning into each other's thought and feeling states. The approach elaborates subjective experience to facilitate interpersonal understanding, integrating important concepts from the fields of attachment theory and reflective function (Fonagy *et al.*, 1991) with these more traditional therapies. It can be used as a stand-alone treatment or as an extension to existing family approaches, enriching the work, we hope, for the ultimate benefit of children and families.

As well as trying to introduce a new perspective on working with families, the MBT-F team takes an innovative approach to manualization. The system we use is web based and uses new, freely available software called TiddlyWiki, which runs in existing web browsers and offers a range of advantages over conventional paper (or even other digital) formats. The manual can easily be searched and is automatically indexed. Material is connected thematically and can be sorted and grouped in almost limitless ways; so that finding a specific piece of material is generally fast (the word 'wiki' comes from the Maori word for 'quick'). Furthermore, when viewed online, the manual will be found to contain a range of streaming video clips of role plays conducted by the MBT-F team, demonstrating specific techniques or aspects of the therapeutic stance as described below. (See also Chapter 9, where the process of tiddly-manualing is described in more detail.)

As the MBT-F manual is freely available (see http://tiddlymanuals.com), we have not tried to summarize the whole model in this chapter, nor do we systematically introduce each of the main components of the work. Instead, we want to give a flavour of some of the key elements of our way of working and describe some of the debates and questions that have arisen for us as we have developed the work.

Introducing the mentalizing stance: the first session

From the beginning of the first meeting, the therapist is aiming to encourage family members to consider the relational aspects of their situation and to both assess the family's current capacity to mentalize and help them see how promoting this capacity may be of value to them. This is established in the first few minutes by asking each person not to say who *they* are, but to introduce the *person next to them* and to say a few words about that person. In this way each family member is encouraged to think about others and to consider relationships from the outset. It is also usually a light-hearted way of opening, with family members searching for the 'best' descriptions, not infrequently prompting laughter or surprise. For example, one child recently chose to introduce her mother by describing how important it was for her to have time in the bathroom in the morning without being disturbed. After getting over her initial embarrassment, the mother was able to be curious about why this would be a fact that her daughter would choose to pick out about her. Some of the emerging information can be picked up later by the therapist; and indeed in this case this insight into a detail of family life led to some important exploration of family dynamics and was a first taste for the family of what it means to 'see oneself as others see you' – a crucial aspect of the capacity to mentalize.

Once family members have introduced each other and given the therapist a sense of who is in the family (sometimes including important people who are not in the room), the next phase concerns itself with exploring what has brought the family to therapy. Again, we find it most useful to start by asking the youngest person in the room to say why they think the family came. This 'inquisitive stance' encompasses enquiries which are respectful, curious and tentative, and emphasizes the importance that the therapist places on trying to understand the feelings and perspectives of others.

It is possible to begin to draw the family's attention to possible patterns of interaction at this stage; for example if a mother interrupts her youngest son to answer for him; or if one member of the family seems to take a back seat whilst the others actively engage with the task. However, often it is best to hear the problem definition from each family member, finishing with the parent/s. The key challenge of holding the balance between letting the natural family interactions flow and intervening will be described in more detail later.

Once all family members have spoken about their understanding of the reason for coming, the therapist can ask various members: 'So what do you make of what your father/grandmother/brother/daughter has said? Do you see it the same way?' The ease or difficulty with which the family is able to do this is also important information for the therapist, who is starting to build a picture of areas of strength and vulnerability in regard to the family's capacity to mentalize. The therapist needs to be able to monitor his or her own thoughts and feelings during this initial engagement period whilst aiming to generate a 'safe and sensitive interpersonal environment' (Fonagy *et al.*, 2011: 104).

From here, the first session usually progresses to discussion about the context and history of the difficulties, including the relationship between family members and individual hopes and desires for therapy outcomes. As in some systemic models, the therapist also focuses on the 'exceptions' to the symptoms, namely when they were mild or absent, and each family member is asked to describe what happened and what each did and thought when 'things were better'. This can be especially helpful for families who have become very organized around a particular problem. With one family, for example, who came to the service because of concern that their nine-year-old son was 'always violent', it was an important step to be able to think about times when he wasn't violent and what was going on for him at those times. Absolute statements ('he's always like that' or 'she just does it to hurt me') are often good indicators of a non-mentalizing stance. So helping families to see exceptions to the rule is again an important aspect of promoting the family's reflective capacity.

In turn, families are also likely to be curious about what they are going to be doing in sessions. Opinion varies within our team regarding the utility of explicitly using the 'M word' in the first meeting. Some find it helpful to introduce the word 'mentalizing', but others try to find different ways to explain the concept. For example, one therapist working with a teenage girl who was staying out late and putting herself in risky situations explained our approach near the end of the first session by saying:

> 'We have been thinking about what might have been going on in Sarah's mind that helps explain why she had to argue so hard to be allowed to stay out late. What you've just been doing is a really good example of a key skill that we use to help us get along with people, and it's the one that we really try to concentrate on in our work here. Surprisingly enough there isn't an existing word for the skill we're trying to practise here, even though we all kind of know about it and we even know a bit about which parts of our brain do this job. So, instead we sometimes use a new word – we call this "making-sense-of-why-a-person-is-behaving-this-way-by-imagining-what-is-going-on-in-their-mind" – **mentalizing.**'

Talking with the family to enable a shared understanding of the approach is a crucial part of making sure that the therapist is explicit with the family about the position they are taking. It allows the therapist to demonstrate openness about sharing his or her own thought processes whilst inviting family members to explore their own.

Holding the balance

Within the MBT-F manual, a key component of the therapist's stance is holding the balance and this primarily refers to the tension between observing the natural interactions within a family and intervening to promote change.

Holding the balance also refers to the active attempt to sustain a balance between a range of other dialectics: for instance, between *thinking* and *feeling*, between *action* and *reflection*, or between *implicit* mentalizing and *explicit* mentalizing. Implicit mentalizing happens automatically, may not involve much conscious awareness and needs a certain amount of affect to stimulate it, whilst explicit mentalizing is typified by a conscious and curious stance which can be overwhelmed and negated by high affect. Put in another way, the holding the balance principle emphasizes that mentalizing is not a capacity that one seeks to sustain continuously: Constant attempts to mentalize oneself or others would be unsustainable and intolerable, extinguishing spontaneity and serendipity. Instead, it is a function whose balanced, judicious and adaptive use at those times when it is needed is (to plunder Donald Winnicott's well-known phrase) *good enough.*

Imagine Johnny, a seven-year-old boy, starts to run across a busy road. In such a moment, it would not be helpful for Johnny's father to stand on the pavement reflecting on what thoughts or feelings in his child may have led to him choosing that particular time to cross the road; instead, immediate action to catch Johnny is necessary. Once returned to the safety of the pavement, it might then be appropriate to check out how Johnny is feeling and also explain why Daddy was shouting at him. However, given the high emotion generated by such an event, it is likely that further discussion, tailored according to Johnny's age and level of understanding, will also be needed when both parties are feeling calmer.

In the therapy, it is the therapist's task to help the family make sense of what feelings are experienced by each family member, as well as highlighting the ways in which miscommunication or misunderstanding (or lack of understanding) of these feelings may lead to interactions that maintain family problems.

In practice, this requires the therapist to strike a very careful balance between allowing the family to interact naturally, simply observing well-worn cycles of non-mentalizing interactions, or indeed actively eliciting habitual and 'normal' family interactions around problematic issues, as well as being directive and intervening at critical moments when necessary. This presents challenges for the therapist in terms of thinking through how to effectively work with families. How much does the therapist need to let the family interactions flow in order to understand the family relationships better and how much does the therapist need to intervene to promote time to pause and reflect with the family and enhance the family's mentalizing about one another?

We would like to share our thinking about some of the factors that may help us hold the balance with different and potentially difficult family interactions. We have found it helpful, in both our individual and team supervision, to begin by considering one's own therapeutic stance; whilst some are more inclined to sit back and observe for some time, others would describe themselves as interventionists, quick to pick up on patterns within families and comment to promote change.

We can also be influenced differently by our family 'scripts' and position in our family of origin (Byng-Hall, 1995). We might ask ourselves how we think others might describe us in our professional role. Or, as a truly multidisciplinary team, including those with psychiatry, psychotherapy, clinical psychology and family therapy backgrounds, whether our training encouraged us to sit back and reflect or to intervene quickly. When thinking about the wider context, we acknowledge the short, fixed-term nature of the particular service we offer, which might lend itself to increasing our desire to move quickly, while being curious about how we might be different if sessions were offered on a longer term basis.

These reflections may offer some sense of positioning in relation to this notion of holding the balance. It can also be helpful to think through situations in which our 'buttons' may be pressed by a family moving us either way on the observation to intervention continuum. For example, one therapist noted that in response to parents being highly critical of their children, she was quickly prompted into action to ask the parents to reflect on how their child may be hearing this criticism rather than observing and waiting to see how other family members may respond to this communication between the parent and the child. Another therapist, however, felt comfortable to wait and see how the family responded, and would then pick up on the pattern that developed within and between different family members.

Having considered some of the factors that impact on our own capacity to hold the balance, it is then helpful to consider the reciprocal loop in which families may engage with us. For example, a family came to MBT-F wanting help to manage their conflictual family relationships. The family comprised a single parent mother with three teenage daughters who pushed boundaries. Mum felt unsupported and overwhelmed and her daughters said their mum had no time for them and always 'nagged'.

At the initial meeting everybody talked at once, interrupted one another and disagreed and tensions quickly escalated. Although one might try in an initial meeting to hold a balance between observing and intervening, given the family's presentation, early intervention was required to promote some room for simply listening. Here we saw that the level of affect in the room tended to rise so quickly that all explicit mentalizing tended to be overwhelmed. When the sense of threat is too great, and the attachment system is activated, the capacity to mentalize typically suffers (Luyten *et al.*, 2009). What was needed was intervention to slow down the speed of exchange and to allow mentalizing to come back 'on-line'.

In the case of this quick-to-rise family, using a 'pause and review' technique to slow down interactions, the therapist invited the family to replay what had happened in the initial few minutes, in order to support building a shared understanding of their experience. The family responded well and began to listen to one another once some structure had been provided. Initially the therapist suggested using a ball, where only the person with the ball could speak, which enabled turn-taking and active listening to take place.

Over time the ball was no longer needed and the family members were more able to take turns. As they became more interested and curious about the different perspectives of each family member, they were better able to pay attention to one another and decided on some plans to share some of the family tasks which had previously caused considerable friction. The daughters had talked with their mother about her not having time for them and mum became tearful and sad about her daughters' experience. This demonstration from mum of hearing and understanding her daughters led the daughters to begin to think about how much their mum did want to have a relationship with them, and to begin to become curious and empathic to her fear that they were going to grow up and distance themselves from her, as she had done herself with her own mother when she was a teenager. From the other side, mum began to see that each of her daughters (in different ways) did want her to give them a bit more space and independence, but that didn't mean they were rejecting her.

As each member of the family began to see the world from each other's perspectives, they became more supportive to each other and this translated into action. They decided to find some more time together as a family; and mum also began to feel more comfortable about giving each of them certain degrees of independence. At the sixth session review one of the daughters explained, 'we just don't shout so much anymore'.

With another family, where a mother and her nine-year-old son spoke freely about their concern about his anxiety (the boy was very preoccupied with thoughts about terrible accidents that might happen to those he loved), the therapist took a step back and listened to the discussion. It initially appeared that they were excellent 'mentalizers', talking together about how difficult a recent separation had been. After three sessions, however, their concerns remained exactly the same. It took a supervisory intervention to see that a helpful balance was not being held here. There was no change in perspective occurring and instead a pattern of well-mannered pseudo-mentalizing was being observed. In this case, whilst there were examples of apparent thoughtfulness, the interaction between mother and son lacked the essential features of genuine mentalization, such as curiosity and perspective taking (acceptance that the same thing can look very different from different perspectives). Instead, thoughts and feelings in others or the self were only recognized as long as they were consistent with the individual's self interest or preferences. In one sense, and in contrast to the family described earlier, the family's patterned responses here served to keep almost all affect out of the room, so that true mentalizing was not 'required' as it might otherwise have been. In this case, activities to re-enact difficult times were designed. The point was to foster sufficient real affect in the room, stimulating the need for implicit mentalizing and moving from a kind of *pretend mode* (Fonagy & Target, 1996) to real explicit mentalizing.

For the worker in the room, this pattern was hard to see at the time. Perhaps this is because of the pressure that such apparently well-mannered behaviour placed upon the therapist (mentalizing approaches would not routinely use the notion of projective identification, but this is another way of explaining what happened). The team in group supervision were insulated from this affect, and were thus more able to mentalize and suggest contingent actions that addressed the situation.

Noticing when families are finding it difficult to make sense of themselves and other people is just as important as highlighting and reinforcing positive mentalizing. For example, when a parent has correctly interpreted how their child might have been feeling when they told a lie about why they weren't home on time the therapist deliberately marks this, for example, by saying: 'I would just like to stop for a second and hear again what dad just had to say because from the smile on your daughter's face, I think you might have guessed how she was feeling.' This can then be checked out with both the daughter and her father and understanding about how he managed to get it right 'this time' can be developed. Then other perspectives can be considered: Did other family members have that same idea? How would they know that she was feeling like that?

Holding the balance is thus an important process of attuning to the family's needs, and MBT-F offers some techniques to facilitate this. These need to be used within the context of an attuned therapeutic relationship, considering where it is most helpful to hold the balance within each individual family and taking into account factors which influence your own capacity as a therapist to hold the balance.

There are of course times when one doesn't get it right, but this too provides an example for everyone to work together to figure out what happened. This will now be considered in the context of the MBT-F loop.

The MBT-F loop

The MBT-F loop (Figure 5.1) is a framework that allows therapists to structure sessions, or at least parts of sessions, to best support both their

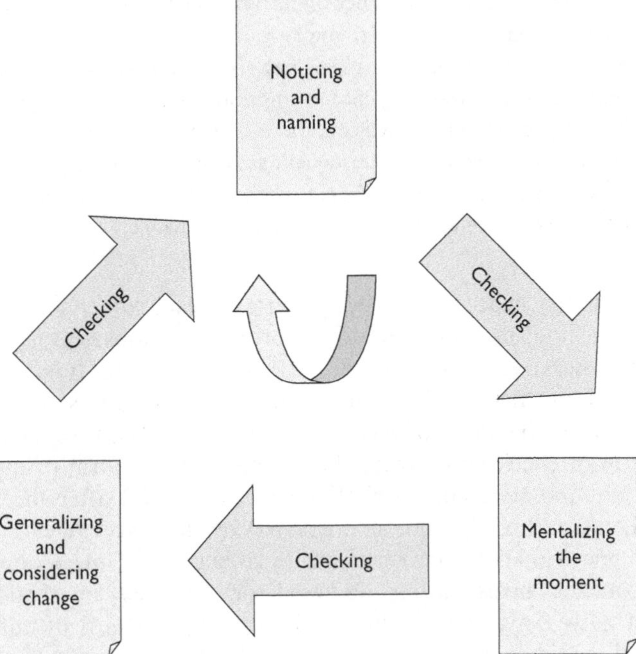

Figure 5.1 The MBT-F loop

own and the family's mentalizing. This provides a route map that can be followed.

These steps are not a simple cycle, but are better conceived of as a spiral; a return to a previous step is never quite the same, as this can only occur in the context of shared experiences and learning that were not present at the first pass. At each or at any step it is possible to use specific mentalizing techniques which aim to stimulate mentalizing within the family.

To explain the usefulness of the MBT-F loop, the model is presented here in a linear fashion, starting from how the therapist uses his process observation(s) of intra-family interactions and/or communication exchanges and how he feeds this back to the family, in an attempt to activate reflexive process in each family member. In practice the MBT-F loop is much more fluid and encourages the creative use of links.

An 11-year-old girl attended with her mother regarding their concerns about the daughter's selective eating. Anya reported struggling with her mother's expectations that now she was at secondary school she should 'suddenly' be eating a wide range of foods that she hadn't before. In this case, both parties were able to 'notice and name' the pattern that appeared at mealtimes with both parties feeling anxious which would lead to Anya refusing to eat. Anya's mother's anxiety would then turn to frustration which meant she would most often end up shouting.

Anya, showing her capacity to reflect on her mother's mind, likened the problem to her mother's attempts to give up smoking. They were able to form a shared understanding of the challenges of changing patterns of behaviour, especially when it was perceived that there were significant emotional 'costs' to change that others had not fully comprehended (mentalizing the moment).

From this they were able to use subsequent sessions to think together about how they would like mealtimes to be different, each choosing one small step towards doing things differently (generalizing and considering change).

As part of the process of making sense of each other's thoughts and feelings, 'checking' provides several important functions and is an integral part of the iterative nature of the MBT-F approach. It is a powerful enactment of the therapist's stance, it confirms the limits of our 'mind-reading', affirms the value of mentalizing and enables us to make links.

One form of checking is where the therapist uses a form of questioning named 'Columbo style curiosity' (Fowler *et al.*, 1995) after the approach used by Lieutenant Columbo, as portrayed by the actor Peter Falk in the American television detective series of the same name. Thus, Columbo-style curiosity means investigating observed or reported interactions in a somewhat naive way, which acknowledges the opaqueness of minds: 'This may sound stupid, but can I just check this? I think I might have got this completely wrong, but do you mind if I . . .?'

If the therapist has indeed got it 'wrong', then a discussion can take place about how that happened. Further checking can then take place about how the therapist might know that he or she had misunderstood someone or how other family members would know, for example, if dad didn't agree with something mum was saying.

This principle of checking out one's own understanding by actively showing an interest in the perspectives of others is something that runs through the work in our team. We try to make use of such monitoring processes, both in the moment and at periodic points in the therapy, such as the mid-therapy review session. This attitude also informs our attitude to evidence and evaluation, which we consider an essential element of the work we do.

Initial evaluation of MBT-F

Whilst continually considering our individual reflections on the families we see, we also invite everyone entering the MBT-F service to take part in a research study designed to measure treatment effectiveness. We are nearing the end of this study, which is naturalistic in design and involves the collection of questionnaire data from children, parents and therapists. We see this monitoring of the service as an important part of the mentalization model itself, within which feedback and seeing things from the other's perspective is crucial.

We use a number of measures within the study,[2] including the Strengths and Difficulties Questionnaire (SDQ; Goodman, 1999), the Health of the Nation Outcome Scales for Children and Adolescents (HoNOSCA; Gowers *et al.*, 1999) and the Children's Global Assessment Scale (CGAS; Shaffer *et al.*, 1983).

Our initial findings from the parent-report SDQ suggest that MBT-F, as a specialist intervention, leads to a statistically significant reduction in behavioural and emotional difficulties in children and young people, as reported by their parents. When we look specifically at the 'emotional symptoms' subscale of the parent-report SDQ, our results show that, in line with the aims of the service and also with other studies of therapeutic effectiveness (Diamond & Josephson, 2005), children showed statistically significant improvement in their emotional well-being over the period during which they received MBT-F and for up to one year later.

Thinking more broadly, the 'impact' supplement of the SDQ allows us to gauge the chronicity of a child's difficulties, the distress and social

2 Although it would have been interesting to do so, we do not currently use any of the specific measures of mentalizing capacity that were described in Chapter 3, as this would place a higher 'burden of assessment' on the families involved than we felt was appropriate in this kind of naturalistic evaluation.

impairment that they cause for him or her, and the burden that these difficulties puts on others. Over the course of MBT-F, parents report an overall reduction in the impact that such difficulties have on both individual and family functioning. Given the relatively small sample size (n=30) we must be cautious, but the results thus far are promising.

Our therapist-report measures, including the HoNOSCA and the CGAS, are completed after the first therapy session and then at the final therapy session. Analysis of the variance of the scores pre- and post-treatment (n=68) showed that for both measures, we recorded a highly significant improvement over time and that this is extremely unlikely to be due to chance alone. So, from the therapist's perspective, it would appear that there are clear changes in the social and emotional functioning of the child which was initially causing parental concern.

We also ask families about their experiences of MBT-F using the Experience of Service Questionnaire (ESQ) that was devised by the Commission for Health Improvement (Attride-Stirling, 2002). Some families, where perhaps the difficulties had been more longstanding, did report that they wished the service was available for more than ten sessions, while others noted that the sessions had offered enough support at that time. One family, where both parents and their three children attended, gave the following feedback, which is fairly representative of other responses we received:

> The problems have been seen from a different angle or perspective, [our therapist] has been very understanding, caring and we have been given many new tips on how to do things differently.

The three children commented that the therapist listened to them, that it was a calm environment and that the therapy 'was really good because we played games to express our feelings'.

Conclusion

Just as we ask families to 'play' with different perspectives, we hope this chapter has given some examples about the ways that we, as therapists and MBT-F team members, also play with different ways of working using a mentalizing framework to support families in difficulty.

Overall, our reflections on our experiences and the encouraging early results provide evidence that supports MBT-F as effective in reducing both individual emotional distress and the impact that this has on families. We continue to seek innovations to our service, including developing adaptations for working with looked after and adopted children, striving to continuously evaluate our practice and disseminating our work through published work, presentations and regular training events.

We feel strongly that the development of a relatively short-term family treatment that builds on the key principles of mentalization is a valuable addition to mental health services with children and young people.

References

Attride-Stirling, J. (2002). *Development of methods to capture users' views of child and adolescent mental health services in clinical governance reviews*. London: Commission for Health Improvement.

Bateman, A., & Fonagy, P. (2004). Mentalization based treatment of borderline personality disorder. *Journal of Personality Disorder*, 18, 36–51.

Byng-Hall, J. (1995). *Rewriting family scripts*. New York: Guilford Press.

Cecchin, G. (1987). Hypothesising, circularity and neutrality revisited: An invitation to curiosity. *Family Process*, 26, 405–413.

de Shazer, S. (1982). *Patterns of brief therapy: An ecosystemic approach*. New York: Guilford Press.

Diamond, G. S., & Josephson, A. (2005). Family based treatment research: A 10-year update. *Journal of American Academy of Child and Adolescent Psychiatry*, 44(9), 872–887.

Donovan, M. (2009). Reflecting processes and reflective functioning: Shared concerns and challenges in systemic and psychoanalytic therapeutic practice. In C. Flaskas & D. Pocock (Eds.), *Systems and psychoanalysis. Contemporary integrations in family therapy*. London: Karnac.

Fearon, P., Target, M., Sargent, J., Williams, L. L., McGregor, J., Bleiberg, E., *et al.* (2006). Short-term mentalization and relational therapy (SMART): An integrative family therapy for children and adolescents. In J. G. Allen & P. Fonagy (Eds.), *Handbook of mentalization-based treatment*. Chichester: Wiley.

Fonagy, P., & Target, M. (1996). Playing with reality I: Theory of mind and the normal development of psychic reality. *International Journal of Psychoanalysis*, 77, 217–233.

Fonagy, P., Steele, H., Moran, G., Steele, M., & Higgitt, A. (1991). The capacity for understanding mental states: The reflective self in parent and child and its significance for security of attachment. *Infant Mental Health Journal*, 13, 200–217.

Fonagy, P., Bateman, A., & Bateman, A. (2011). Commentary: The widening scope of mentalizing: A discussion. *Psychology and Psychotherapy: Theory, Research and Practice*, 84, 98–110.

Fowler, D., Garety, P., & Kuipers, E. (1995). *Cognitive behaviour therapy for psychosis: Theory and practice*. Chichester: Wiley.

Goodman, R. (1999). The extended version of the Strengths and Difficulties Questionnaire as a guide to child psychiatric caseness and consequent burden. *Journal of Child Psychology and Psychiatry*, 40(5), 791–801.

Gowers, S. G., Harrington, R. C., Whitton, A., Lelliott, P., Beevor, A., Wing, J., *et al.* (1999). Brief scale for measuring the outcomes of emotional and behavioural disorders in children: Health of the Nation Outcome Scales for Children and Adolescents (HoNOSCA). *British Journal of Psychiatry*, 174(5), 413–416.

Larner, G. (2000). Towards a common ground in psychoanalysis and family therapy: On knowing not to know. *Journal of Family Therapy*, 22, 61–82.

Luyten, P., Mayes, L., Fonagy, P., & Van Houdenhove, B. (2009). The interpersonal regulation of stress. Unpublished manuscript.

Minuchin, S. (1974). *Families and Family Therapy*. Cambridge, MA: Harvard University Press.

Pocock, D. (2009). Working with emotional systems: Four new maps. In C. Flaskas & D. Pocock (Eds.), *Systems and psychoanalysis. Contemporary integrations in family therapy*. London: Karnac.

Rober, P. (1999). The therapist's inner conversation in family therapy practice: Some ideas about the self of the therapist, therapeutic impasse and the process of reflection. *Family Process*, 38, 209–228.

Sandler, J. (1976). Countertransference and role responsiveness. *International Review of Psychoanalysis*, 3, 43–47.

Selvini Palazzoli, M., Boscolo, L., Cecchin, G., & Prata, G. (1980). Hypothesizing-circularity-neutrality: Three guidelines for the conductor of the session. *Family Process*, 19, 3–12.

Shaffer, D., Gould, M. S., Brasic, J., Ambrosini, P., Fisher, P., Bird, H. R., *et al.* (1983). A Children's Global Assessmemt Scale (CGAS). *Archives of General Psychiatry*, 40, 1228–1231.

Chapter 6

Mentalization-based therapies with adopted children and their families

Nicole Muller, Lidewij Gerits and Irma Siecker

Introduction

The development of most adopted children progresses smoothly. However, if concerns do emerge, and their families seek out help from child and adolescent mental health services (CAMHS), it often appears as if the children's problems are linked to their difficult start in life. Therapeutic services offered to these families need to be aware of this and adapt their services accordingly, paying particular attention to the specific vulnerabilities that adopted children and their families may have.

This chapter will give an account of our team's work with the families of adopted children using mentalization-based treatment for families (MBT-F), often in combination with MBT play therapy for the young child, or MBT group therapy for adopted adolescents. It will include a description of our team's work and express our optimism at being able to support and help adoptive families overcome the complex problems they encounter.

The impact of early experience on adopted children

How well children survive physical, emotional or mental trauma depends a great deal on the quality of the attachment relationships in their actual lives. Unresolved trauma can have a huge impact on the attachment behaviour of adopted children towards their caregivers. There is a great deal of debate currently around whether the negative effects of early traumatic experiences can be overcome and if those suffering unresolved trauma will ever be able to feel the love and care of others or experience what it means to be loved.

Different long-term developmental consequences in the way adopted children are able to relate to themselves and others have been observed. They depend on the nature of the pre-placement conditions, a child's vulnerabilities and strengths, and the circumstances of the family that adopts the child. Many adopted children lived in orphanages during the key developmental period for learning to form and maintain attachment relationships. With the exception of those placed in adoptive families at birth, most adopted children have experienced neglect, and some abuse, either alone or in combination with neglect (Dozier & Rutter, 2008).

Recent research by Van den Dries (2010) showed that adopted children, between 11 and 16 months old, undergo a major developmental leap in specific areas, such as mental development and physical growth, in the first half year after adoption. A meta-analysis also revealed that adoptees have a higher risk of disorganized attachment relationships than non-adopted children (Van den Dries *et al.*, 2009). At the same time, the risk of disorganized attachment in adopted children is the highest for children who grew up in institutions. Van den Dries (2010) also found that children who are adopted after their first birthday are less securely attached; whereas children who are adopted before their first birthday are as securely attached as non-adopted children.

It can be inferred that attachment insecurity and emotional and behavioural difficulties are more likely to increase as a result of adoption after six months of age or following early abuse or deprivation (Johnson, 2000, 2002). Prolonged institutionalization presents a set of risks leading to social deprivation and reduced stimulation of sensory, cognitive and linguistic development (Johnson, 2000). This may help to explain why adoptees and their families have had higher than expected rates of referral to mental health services (Brodzinsky *et al.*, 1998).

Adoptees are also over-represented in the group of children with attention deficit hyperactivity disorder (ADHD) and disruptive behavioural disorders such as conduct disorder (Brodzinsky *et al.*, 1998). They are also four times as likely as non-adoptees to have a learning disability (Brodzinsky *et al.*, 1993). Several studies have found that severe attention disorder is related to disorganized attachment. This phenomenon has been observed in Romanian orphans who, not having benefited from a reassuring attachment figure, had difficulty focusing attention properly due to high stress levels (Kreppner *et al.*, 2001). When non-adopted and adopted teenagers were compared to each other, the adoptees revealed greater difficulty with socio-emotional functioning during adolescence (Johnson, 2000, 2002).

Challenges for adoptive parents

In a securely attached mother and child dyad, the child's experiences are repeatedly mentalized by the parents. As a result, the child learns that there are other minds with intentions, and that the child has his own intentions which may differ from the intentions of others. This capacity enables the child to plan, anticipate and learn to express feelings and thoughts, to regulate emotions, to reflect on experiences and describe these representations (Fonagy *et al.*, 2002). This interaction is primarily unconscious and implicit.

Jemerin (2004) describes the normal interaction between a mentalizing parent and latency children. The parent is usually able to endure the feelings of the child, can give a representation through marked mirroring and can reframe the situation or feeling – at least for most of the time. In turn, the child can successfully profit from this type of interaction because of the repetition of all the non-verbal experiences within the parent–child relationship, which helps the child feel understood and acknowledged. Adopted children often lack such experiences in their early lives. This can inhibit their ability to feel understood, retarding this specific aspect of their emotional development, as well as making it hard for them to make use of the representations or reframing of a parent. The parent and child do not yet know each other's story or speak each other's language. For this reason, adoptive parents and their adopted children often struggle to understand each other. The spontaneous and intuitive reaction of most parents toward a child may not occur because the child reacts in a seemingly incomprehensible way. Furthermore, the adopted child is often not capable of providing words for their feelings or meaning for their behaviour.

All latency children depend during their development on the reflective functioning capabilities of their parents (Jemerin, 2004). Without assistance from the adoptive parent and/or therapist to mentalize, the adopted child cannot connect or transfer memories encoded in implicit non-verbal awareness to explicit verbal conscious memories. Adoptive parents often have difficulty in decoding or reflecting on the (psychopathological) behaviour of their children because of the non-shared pre-adoption period, or due to the lack of information about birth parents and the circumstances surrounding conception and birth. Moreover, the attachment relationship between the child and adoptive parent is still in development and remains vulnerable and often unpredictable for each of them.

MBT-F with adopted children and their families

One of the goals of MBT-F is to increase the effort made by adopted children's parents and teachers to understand the child's behaviour (Allen *et al.*, 2008; Muller & Bakker, 2009). During MBT-F sessions with parents, families and schoolteachers, we share a great deal of our knowledge about attachment, trauma and mentalization in order to help those we work with gain a better understanding of the problems involved in each situation. It is beneficial for those around the child to understand the child's behavioural and emotional problems as both a reflection of biological susceptibility and as an effort to cope and adapt to an insecure situation. For example, our team invites children and parents to consider how a baby in an orphanage might find ways to survive and learn to ask for care and attention. We explain how every child seeks mechanisms for self-consolation and tries to gain a sense of control over her circumstances. However, these early coping behaviours are not always suitable in their present situation.

Further goals of MBT-F are to increase each family member's understanding of each other, and improve the attunement between them. We try to stimulate curiosity in the feelings of each member of the family, the thoughts connected to these feelings, and the manner in which they are expressed and understood (Allen *et al.*, 2008). It is difficult for a child or parent to mentalize about the behaviour and feelings of oneself or others in moments of great distress or emotion, which has a direct effect on one's sense of feeling connected to others. Therefore we search for the stressful situations that trigger or cause a child or parent to lose contact (Muller & ten Kate, 2008).

Sometimes adoptive parents really struggle to understand their children, which can have a huge effect on the way they think about themselves as parents or in the way they see and understand their adopted child. A parent's capacity to make sense of both their own and their child's mental states plays a crucial role in helping the child (Fonagy *et al.*, 2002). Presumably, it is a parent's capacity to tolerate and regulate their own internal, affective experiences that allows them to tolerate and regulate these experiences in their child (Slade, 2010).

During an MBT-F session with the parents of an adopted son named David, 12 years old, the mother tended to speak for her son and appeared to know exactly what he thought and felt, as if the mother's internal state had merged with her interpretation of the supposed internal state of the child. This was very understandable because the boy had such difficulty with recognizing his emotions, thoughts and actions. David had lived in terribly neglectful conditions with his biological mother, who had died when he was four years old. He continuously kept on idealizing his 'fantastic birthmother', making her drawings for 'the most lovely mother on earth'. The mother spoke of the feelings of David as if she knew he missed his birthmother every day and how she could understand this because she felt her deep love for her own mother. However, in talking with her the therapist asked how she really felt about these drawings and what she really felt towards the mother of David. She then realized she felt rejected by David, because she tried so hard to be the second best mother in the world. And with the help of her husband she also realized that deep down inside she was so angry at the mother of David for what she didn't do for this wonderful child.

After we had acknowledged the mother's attempt to understand her son, we could start a new session by asking David what he thought about his birthmother and his adoptive mother. We were trying to get him more involved in thinking about himself and attempting to help his mother learn that it is impossible to know precisely what another person thinks or feels. David became more involved as the session progressed. This was also possible because the mother understood her own feelings and therefore could tolerate his ambivalent emotions and loyalties about mothers.

The parents were further stimulated through the process of reflecting on the possible consequences of not fully understanding their child and their own feelings, and how their diminished curiosity about their son's feelings and thoughts might make him feel. It seemed that the mother had fears of losing her son in the future, making her anxious at times. David was surprised to hear about his mother's anxieties.

It is very important to support the parents of adopted children. Their child's intense behaviours can leave adoptive parents full of doubt about their ability to parent. This might lead to feelings of inadequacy or rejection on the parent's behalf, which unbalances the relationships within the family. Parents may initially have had elevated expectations about parenting or an idealized picture of adoption. If so, being confronted with a different reality can be painful.

Parents will often report that they are having trouble dealing with rejection and the lack of emotional reciprocity from their child, which can result in feelings of rejection and insecurity on the part of the adoptive parents. We try to help them become aware of their own expectations of motherhood and fatherhood over the course of MBT-F. They often face feelings of disappointment and helplessness in their inability to alleviate their children's problems.

During one session with the parents of three adopted siblings from Ghana – the youngest named Sammy, with severe behavioural and emotional problems – the father talked about feeling burned out due to the fact that he could not get a grip on his son. The therapist discussed what this meant for him. The father became very emotional and talked about his feelings of powerlessness and his belief that his son didn't want to be with them. This brought Sammy's father back to the time they first welcomed Sammy and his two brothers into the family. As a toddler, Sammy cried and cried and would not be consoled. His parents felt both powerless and hopeless during this period, as well as feeling rejected by Sammy. The father continued to re-experience these emotions from time to time, and interpreted the behaviour of his child as a rejection, personally aimed at him. The therapist accepted the father's feelings at face value and tried to understand the pain of this rejection as Sammy's father felt it. After exploring the father's feelings of alienation from his son, we also searched for new perspectives on the intentions behind Sammy's behaviour.

By asking clients to tell personal stories about their lives, we are trying to help them deal with inner conflicts and tensions. Stories combine content with context and help people to adapt to change (Ochs & Capps, 2001). Autobiographical continuity is part of a person's self-representation: it is the capacity to remember oneself in the past and to experience the continuity of internal states, in spite of one's changes (Bleiberg, 2001). Adoptees and adoptive parents might have multiple fantasized stories about the conception, birth and previous circumstances of the adopted child. These may be both unconscious and conscious, and at times incompatible. A central challenge is constructing a coherent narrative about the adoptee and his family that involves both the birth family and the adoptive family. We help adopted children to explore their experiences in current relationships as well as their narrative about past relationships through questions such as: 'Do you feel at home?' 'What does the word *home* mean to you?' 'In what way do you feel that your family belongs together?' 'What does the word family mean to you?' 'How often do you think about your birth parents?' 'What do you call them?' Such questions help adoptive families to discover both experienced relationships and the sense of self and other, thereby increasing their capacity to learn to mentalize explicitly and helping the adopted child to tell a coherent 'what makes me me' story.

Adoptive parents frequently find it difficult to set clear limits for their children. Many adopted children have suffered rejection, violence and neglect early in life and understandably parents – and psychotherapists – want to make up for this misfortune either out of sympathy or sensitivity to the child's longing for unconditional love. Parents often worry that their adopted child will experience parental anger as something frightening or rejecting. On the other hand, some of these children have extreme behavioural problems and can be very violent towards others, demolishing furniture and stealing money or food.

Our team encourages parents to think about their child in terms of the child's internal experiences, rather than in terms of their behaviour. MBT-F is indeed about identifying with the child's and parents' feelings and thoughts, rather than their actions (Slade, 2010). However, this can be tricky for some adoptive parents due to the extreme behaviour their child may exhibit. The aggressive behaviour exhibited by the adoptee is often linked to the existential theme of fear of yet another abandonment, resulting in the persistent testing of the parent–child bond. In other words, not allowing a bond to develop can be understood as favourable to the pain of another abandonment and the renewed sense of powerlessness that arises from not being able to shape one's own life and future. Is it any wonder these children try to control others and direct their own lives in a predictable way?

Violence is nevertheless largely incompatible with the sentiment of attachment to another, and being able to mentalize how aggression distresses a loved one can help adopted children to control their violent outbursts (Bleiberg, 2001). This mentalization process may help adoptees become more aware of the effect of their behaviour on significant others. However, mentalizing about oneself in order to understand the nature of one's own impulses is far from easy. Violent outbursts appear to happen spontaneously, like a disruptive impulse.

What can help an adopted child who sometimes acts so aggressively? Deprived children need loving, caring and curious people around them who are not preoccupied with their own feelings and who can facilitate the adopted child to think about their inner world. This helps the child to stay connected with himself and others, and to find new ways of dealing with painful, anxious and at times devastating emotions. In certain cases, it helps to develop cues that are used to inhibit the disruptive impulses. However, cueing is not always effective or the behaviour may require immediate action; for example, it may be necessary to stop aggressive outbursts in order to keep the home environment safe. The challenge is to find ways in which a parent can bring an end to the aggressive behaviour in a clear and beneficial manner and to set limits without losing contact with their child. Due to both the parents' and their adopted child's tendency towards non-mentalizing reactions, such as running away and not wanting to return home, this can be quite a challenge.

During one MBT-F session, which took place with a family of four children adopted from Brazil, the youngest boy Leo – 14 years old at the time – was in the spotlight. It had already emerged that he had a tendency to become very aggressive and hostile towards his mother at times. Leo's latest outburst had occurred two days previous to this session and was being discussed. The therapist was interested in how the outburst had affected Leo's mother; she was still very emotional about it. She expressed her sadness over the fact that she had turned away from her son during the outburst. She was upset by Leo's cursing and the level of anger that Leo expressed made her fearful of him. She walked away while he was demolishing the furniture in his room. The mother's tension diminished visibly as she expressed her feelings. The therapist then asked Leo what it meant to him to hear that his mother had become afraid of him. He became very sad during this session, as he began to realize the damaging effect his behaviour had had on his relationship with his mother. He apologized to his mother. At this point our team focused on discovering the emotion that had triggered Leo's anger in the first place.

Some parents are so focused on being the best parent possible that they tend to view every mistake as a failure. They do not show their emotions or put their own needs forward. This has a tremendous effect on a parent's reflective functioning and thus on the relationship between them and their children. During MBT-F, therapists will encourage such parents to explore why they find it so hard to set limits. The parent will be supported as they think about the consequences of their behaviour and attitude to themselves, as a parent, and to their children. Parental limit setting can evoke strong feelings in an adopted child, such as anger about the adoption or idealized feelings about biological parents. They may strike out against their adoptive parents and demand to go back to their birthmother. This can be very painful for the adoptive parents and evokes strong feelings in return, limiting the parents' capacity to mentalize. One consequence of the above is an overreaction by the parents, possibly leading to a demanding parenting style, as the parents are also in need of confirmation. MBT-F attempts to enhance the understanding of each other's beliefs and expectations and requires both parents and children to take responsibility when dealing with problems.

The psychotherapist must set clear limits during MBT-F as well, and takes on a directive role during sessions. Non-mentalizing interactions, such as when a parent is full of negativity about current circumstances and wants to use the session to ventilate her frustrations, must be stopped in their tracks. When there is hostility or aggression in the room, we stop this immediately to hold the balance between letting the natural interaction flow, managing the arousal level and intervening to promote change.

The participants in one session, involving 12-year-old adopted twins, were throwing a (soft) ball around the room. The exercise included throwing the ball in an angry way, followed by throwing it in a loving way. When throwing the ball angrily, one of the twins threw the ball hard at her mother's head. The therapist stopped the session immediately and posed non-judgemental questions such as: 'What is happening now?' 'I see a lot of tension in your body – do you notice that?' 'How is mum?' and asking the mum 'What did you experience when you got that ball thrown at you in this way?'

MBT-F therapists should maintain the practice of mentalizing about themselves and their clients during sessions and interdisciplinary staff meetings, because clients will push their buttons as well. We need to acknowledge that these children and their parents can also awake rescue fantasies in ourselves. It is difficult for a therapist to mentalize about her own limits and feelings, as well as the limits and abilities of her organization. Sometimes we have to deal with our own feelings of powerlessness, recognizing that we do not have an answer for everyone and accepting this painful reality.

During interpersonal interactions, mentalization is generally done in an implicit, automatic and non-reflective manner. This implicit learning process is the basis of one's ability to react to non-verbal emotional communication. Explicit mentalizing is enhanced by learning to focus on implicit processes, such as our automatic reactions to others, in the belief that self-awareness can increase (Allen, *et al.*, 2008).

During a MBT-F session with a nine-year-old boy named Chico and his father, the therapist asked Chico to choose music that he associated with the following emotions: happiness, anger, fear and sadness. He chose 'To Make You Feel My Love' by Adèle for sadness. Both Chico and his father became sad, with tears rolling down their cheeks, while listening to the music. The words from the text, 'I would do anything to make you feel my love', were the same words the father would say to Chico during times of great distress. It was very hard for Chico to feel that he is loved when he is, for example, at school, trying to get along with other children. In order to have Chico reflect on this feeling in the here and now, the therapist asked questions such as: 'What makes you sad?' and 'What do you think makes your father sad?'

It can be incredibly hard for some parents to find the courage not only to trust, but also to build on the relationship that exists between them and their children. If parents have the sense that they are central to their children's lives, and are needed for comfort, support and acknowledgement, they will become more confident in their parenting role. The paradox is that adopted children are not always capable of returning affection, and furthermore these same children may even need to be taught how to ask for comfort and support. They may also be unwilling to accept physical contact. The overall effect can leave parents insecure about their role and incapable of building up a critical level of trust within the relationship.

Adopted children who have been traumatized early in life are frequently left with a fragmented representation of self and others and an array of highly disturbing feelings locked away inside. As a result, they will most likely evoke different reactions in people under distinct circumstances. Adopted children will sometimes behave very differently at school than at home and may either incite aggressive reactions from others or seek to blend in and become invisible. Our team has therefore chosen to undertake the expansion of MBT into schools in order to address and ease the school life of adopted children with histories of early trauma.

One goal of this school-based scheme is to make it feasible for classmates to accept the unusual emotional reactions and behaviours of the adopted child. After all, being 'different' can be stigmatizing among children. A second goal is to address cases of splitting phenomena between parents and the school. Under such circumstances, parents generally find it very hard to accept, for example, that their child acts in a threatening manner at school, or conversely that he is quiet and withdrawn in the classroom, when they contend with the opposite behaviour at home. This type of contradictory behaviour can be found in extreme cases of sibling rivalry as well.

According to MBT-F, the point in this situation is to try and comprehend the unusual mental states of early trauma victims in collaboration with the adoptee and her family, as well as attempting to endure the painful circumstances and feelings that surround these mental states for all involved.

Challenges for the adopted child

In our practice, MBT-F has proven to be the most beneficial for adopted children when applied simultaneously with individual MBT play therapy, which addresses and boosts the awareness of inner feelings and thoughts and the explicit mentalization of them. A child therapist regularly attends MBT-F sessions in order to facilitate the child as he tries to understand and explore his present feelings and thoughts. Within the safe and relaxed context of play therapy, themes like ambivalence and loyalty can be explored and used to support the MBT-F sessions.

Feelings of abandonment, loss and uncertainty preoccupy many adoptees during childhood. Due to this characteristic 'existential susceptibility', the therapist can expect certain themes to arise during treatment, in the form of questions, such as: 'Do I have a right to live?' 'Why was I given away?' and 'Do my parents love me?' (Oprell, 2005). This existential susceptibility affects adopted children's capacity to strengthen the attachment relationship with their adoptive parents at a very fundamental level. Children also depend on this same basic attachment level in order to mentalize. It is therefore not surprising that extra support from MBT play therapy is valuable in helping adopted children with (explicit) mentalizing during family therapy.

Mentalizing difficulties can manifest themselves in various ways in adopted children. A child may perceive their own feelings in an egocentric way, under the assumption that the other thinks and feels exactly as they do, making it harder to mentalize about the inner states of others. As a rule, however, adopted children pay little attention to others or their own feelings. For that reason it is very important for adopted children to help them pay attention to their own inner world and help them realize that their inner thoughts and feelings do not necessarily have to match reality.

One striking observation during a therapy session with ten-year-old Jacky was that she often missed non-verbal cues from her parents. At one point her mother joined the therapy session for a few moments. Jacky did not notice that her mother was sad until the therapist pointed it out. She was incapable of imagining what could have upset her mother at this time.

Other adoptive children mentalize about others excessively, displaying a form of hyper-vigilance for the mental states of others. This seems to occur when a child has had to be extremely alert to her surroundings in the past, due to a constant threat of abuse or violence. These children pay too much attention to others and at the same time show too little interest in their own mental states. Furthermore, regardless of their diligence, they appear to misinterpret the mental states of others.

Some of these difficulties can be thought of from a developmental perspective. A child develops a subjective sense of self through the repetition of marked mirroring of the self in the representation of the parents. Many traumatized adopted children have a fragmented sense of self originating in disorganized attachment relationships. Projective identification is one of the mechanisms used by adopted children to externalize their intolerable physical and emotional features. When negative aspects of memories are so intense and frequently present in the parent–child dyad and the parent is no longer capable of regulating the emotions of the child, he may not be able to represent them in a 'detoxified' way, and a defensive and pathological form of projective identification can be the result (Schmeets & Verheugt-Pleiter, 2005). Besides projective identification dissociation also plays an important role in the above context and will be discussed in some detail at this point.

The child's lack of a coherent self is visible and tangible in the fragmentation of time, place and person that adopted children with a history of early trauma tend to exhibit during MBT play sessions. There is often little sense of continuity between an adopted child's behaviour and expressed affect across the range of contexts in the child's life, over a series of MBT play sessions or even within a single session. These children may seem very different during therapy than they do at home or at school. They will not spontaneously tell stories about events in their everyday lives. As a result, the therapeutic setting risks being experienced as an anomaly. Since the variety of behaviours an adoptive family may witness are not always immediately visible to the child's therapist, parental feelings of frustration and uncertainty are common. Alternatively, the therapist may feel a connection with only one part of the child, knowing that much remains unsaid and unseen, no doubt partially due to frequent dissociation. This makes it much harder for a therapist to trust his own intuition, which is especially problematic, as therapists are trained to use their own emotional responses as an instrument to understand the client's inner experiences and their relationship with the client as a tool to foster therapeutic change.

Jacky, eight years old, began therapy because of behavioural problems at home. Her parents often felt used by her and interpreted the purpose of her behaviour overall as self-rewarding. They also worried about her moral development, as she seemed to have no regrets about her aggressive outbursts towards her mother. Within the therapeutic relationship, Jacky came across as extremely insecure and behaved in an overly adaptive way. She appeared to be suppressing all forms of direct aggression. During play, on the other hand, Jacky exhibited a great deal of aggression, but without any real feeling behind the aggressive acts. Her play was repetitive and rigid and displayed little emotion. The therapist noticed that some important emotional themes were present, but still felt little contact with this girl. She found it very hard to stay focused due to the large gap between the explicit and implicit aspects of their relationship.

Recent research has revealed that projective identification is often utilized as a strategy for affect regulation, which in an adaptive way is part of normal development (Schmeets & Verheugt-Pleiter, 2005). However, this mechanism is strongly influenced by events during the first year of life. When negative aspects dominate, a more defensive mechanism arises. Therefore, projective identification, as a defence mechanism, is frequently seen in adopted children. This can cause extreme emotions within the child–adoptive parent relationship – as well as within the child–therapist relationship – and interactions may become susceptible to re-enactment. At the same time, this mechanism is a way for the therapist to get to know the pre-verbal experiences and internal representations of the child (Wallin, 2007). This can only be achieved if the therapist is able to maintain mentalization about his own negative feelings evoked within this relationship. The challenge for the therapist is to set limits that both provide safety and allow contact with the child, while also enabling the therapist to maintain his capacity to mentalize and regulate his own affective states. For example, during seven-year-old Pete's fourth play therapy session, he immediately picked up on a game where he had left it the previous session. The therapist reported as follows:

> The last therapy session Pete had played with the dolls and was focused on taking care of them. This time he started the same play but included me in the game. He wanted me to take over the nurturing of the doll and gave explicit instructions for me how to handle it. As the play went along the instructions became more inappropriate. The baby needed to be held and as I cuddled the baby, Pete made the baby touch me. Gradually this touching became more intrusive. The baby wanted to touch my breasts and he gave me instructions that I had to kiss the baby on his private parts. The play felt really intrusive. Pete was very determined and seemed to have no emotions at all.
>
> I felt this game was getting to me. I was uncomfortable with the role he gave me and I didn't want to do the things he told me to do. I could nonetheless also feel the value of the game, and it seemed to me that Pete was trying to make me feel a specific emotion. As a result, I chose to continue playing and attempted to find a way to deal with my own feelings. One way was to continue but also set limits. I continued to hold the doll but said that I did not want to kiss the doll on his private parts and I prevented Pete, through the doll, from touching my breasts. I stayed in contact with Pete outside the game and talked about reality. This helped me to regulate my own feelings. I also expressed my feelings of awkwardness and that it seemed to me that this kissing and touching is not what an adult should do with a child. I did this from my perspective and from the perspective of the doll without interpreting anything to Pete.

The above example provides a lesson about the role projective identification can play within MBT play therapy, as well as reminding us that setting boundaries is essential both implicitly and explicitly. Children with a disorganized attachment style, who therefore have difficulties with mentalizing, are not attuned to signals indicating the acceptable level of contact between people, and are prone to crossing the personal limits set by others. This pattern will appear in the therapeutic relationship as well. The therapist needs to cope with the adopted child's inappropriate behaviour by mentalizing; for example, by naming the effect the behaviour is having and exploring the interaction. The therapist may be confronted with extreme internal emotions at times, such as those portrayed in the example above. Setting boundaries sensitively then becomes an essential regulatory strategy for both the therapist and the child. Without boundaries, the level of anxiety can become impairing for children (Verheugt-Pleiter, 2008). This seems to be especially true for those who function heavily in the 'psychic equivalence mode', and whose internal and external realities are experienced by them as more or less the same.

Therapeutic challenges in working with loss and the dysregulation of emotions in the adopted child

One of the primary goals of treatment for adopted children is thought to be facilitating the mourning of losses associated with adoption (Nickman, 1985). However Quinodoz (1996) claims that there is no way to mourn something that has not been experienced. Furthermore, according to Pivnick (2010: 16): 'It is possible then, that in the absence of a mentalized image of, or narrative concerning the birth parents, adoptees identify with the non-mentalizable itself, that is, with inefficient cognition or lack of curiosity, as a way of enacting what cannot be found.'

The above theories play a role in illuminating why therapy does not always help adoptees, especially latency children, to mourn what they have lost. At an implicit level, nevertheless, there is always an available narrative about the adoption circumstances that influences functioning in daily life. Adoptees have internal representations of both their biological and their adoptive parents. Even if the child has no background information whatsoever, they will implicitly create a narrative based largely on their fantasies. In these cases, the biological parents become either idealized or are completely rejected. This can manifest in a number of ways, such as behaviour aimed at avoiding another abandonment or possibly 'bad seed' behaviour. One of our clients, Harry, provides an excellent example of the latter. He liked to say: 'My father was a criminal, and ended up in jail, and so will I.'

In object relations theory the confrontation with reality plays an important part. According to Winnicott (1992) it is the good-enough real mother as opposed to the internal idealized mother who helps the child make an increasing differentiation of inner and outer reality. Klein (1975) wrote about the integration of the good and the bad object and the development of a psychic reality distinct from the physical world. In both theories it is crucial that the real parental figures are around to demonstrate the continuity of their love. When an adopted child has not experienced this continuity in the confrontation with reality, due to a lack of continuity in primary caregivers, it can be very difficult for him to learn to deal with ambivalence, thus making it impossible for the child to connect external and internal realities or to bond with an internal representation. Our team has observed adoptive children with such strong ambivalent feelings that they can no longer manage them. This may explain why some adopted children are unable to mentalize explicitly about their birth family's background or mourn over what was lost. Implicitly, these feelings can become part of the therapeutic relationship, as well as of other relationships the child forms.

Another explanation for why it often seems so difficult for adopted children to organize their experiences in a causal-temporal context, and make them a part of their autobiographic self, is because this requires the ability to mentalize explicitly, i.e. at the highest level (Allen *et al.*, 2008). Explicit mentalization about internal representations will consequently be the last phase in therapy, although latency children will not always reach this phase at all. Adolescents, on the other hand, are further developed both cognitively and emotionally. Moreover, identity formation is of itself traditionally associated with adolescence. Consequently, mourning does become an explicit theme within MBT for most adolescent adoptees.

An essential part of MBT play therapy is to learn to regulate emotions. Children adopted after six months of age almost always experience difficulties with this. Some children respond to these problems by functioning largely in the psychic equivalence mode; they experience their internal world as reality and therefore react too quickly to impulses. This leads to poor differentiation between self and other. It is hard for such children to imagine that anyone else could have a state of mind unlike theirs, and accordingly they colour the thoughts and feelings of others with their own emotions. It also leads to extreme changes in affective expression. There is hardly any representation of the external reality's effect on the self, further increasing the difficulty for children who function primarily in the psychic equivalence mode to regulate their own emotions.

Furthermore, these children find it hard to use imagination while they play. This is understandable bearing in mind that fantasy feels like reality to them, often causing overwhelming fear, which they feel unable to regulate (Verheugt-Pleiter, 2008). Such children may mask their lack of imagination with chaotic and impulsive behaviour; for example, in the way they manipulate toys. Therapists can become overwhelmed by the pandemonium surrounding them and will experience difficulty in trying to stay on track while following the child. This type of session can leave a therapist exhausted. The first step then of MBT play therapy is to join in the child's play, searching for ways to share focus and attention, whilst averting superficial contact.

Other adopted children, due to their inability to regulate emotions, seem to us to operate primarily in 'pretend mode' (Fonagy *et al.*, 2002). The opposite reaction to the one described above will occur in this case. These children will have a loose connection between play – external reality – and their internal world. They rarely display congruent emotions and seem to have pulled back from personal relationships, demonstrating little connection to others. Children who operate in a pretend mode generally learn to regulate their own feelings outside of their relationships. Their play can be full of fantasy, and at the same time emotionless and repetitive. It is very hard for a therapist to connect with these children or to connect with their play. There is a temptation to become bored and to lose focus. This is especially true as progress occurs very slowly. The challenge for the therapist is to focus on the search for moments of shared attention and to grasp each in an attempt to be more in tune with the child. Additionally, the therapist must pay special attention to the child's body signals in order to learn more about the emotions the child is experiencing in the here and now. This is even more difficult, owing to the ambiguous signals these children often give out and because children living in a fantasy world can be so out of touch with their own body that they are often unaware of their signals.

For a long time Caroline, 11 years old, repeated the same game every week during MBT play therapy. The game involved a dollhouse that contained two sisters who expressed sibling rivalry through negative and devaluing behaviour. The sisters were very envious of a rich girl who lived next door. This was a typical theme for Caroline, who prized appearance and material possessions. The game however never advanced and it proved impossible to make an explicit connection between the game and Caroline's inner states.

As a result, the first phase of Caroline's therapy was to focus on becoming more alert to Caroline's apparent behavioural changes during therapy – such as suddenly asking a lot of questions – and making her more aware of this behaviour. By learning to recognize these shifts in attention, she was able to start to explore the meaning of them. Caroline was only able to recognize and connect with some of her own feelings of insecurity – and to share them with the therapist – after this first step had been achieved. Caroline's therapist believed that Caroline enjoyed play therapy with her and that the relationship did indeed have some meaning for her. However, since the therapist could not feel much of a connection in this relationship, she often doubted whether she had genuinely connected at all with Caroline.

An important aspect of play therapy is providing a safe space for adopted children with a history of early trauma. Within this sanctuary they can be facilitated to endure their own emotions and learn to represent and regulate them. At times this may require containing a child's overwhelming and chaotic emotions and mirroring them in a marked and more comprehensible way. At other times this means searching for the emotional signals and increasing the sense of protection, so that the child can safely access and share a painful emotion.

As previously mentioned, it can be very hard for adoptive parents to trust the relationship between themselves and their adopted child. This certainly holds true for therapists as well. Therapists can feel as if they are grasping at straws as they attempt to create a bond with certain children. In an attempt to thwart doubts, a therapist must trust their own capabilities and elicit feedback from colleagues and clients. Debriefings with colleagues and feedback from ex-clients, especially clients from a good number of years previously, can help therapists renew their belief in the importance of therapy. A good example of this can be found in the following testimony of one of this chapter's authors:

> During a recent psychotherapy session, 15-year-old Monique told me just how important play therapy had been for her when she was nine. At that time Monique's behavioural problems were extreme, and I often felt insecure about what I was doing. Monique was not able to deal with certain painful issues about herself and was a child that tended to avoid emotions. I often wondered if our time spent on implicit mentalizing was helping her.
>
> Monique had recently asked to return to therapy with me. She reminded me that she had felt acceptance and approval once a week while under my care; I had helped her to open up to herself. Now an adolescent, she had become more curious about herself and wanted to find words to express her pain. She had retained valuable memories of the play therapy sessions we had together, and claimed that she had thought about them frequently over the past six years. She had kept both the therapy sessions and me in mind throughout this period!

Conclusion

Our team's clinical experience affirms that adoptive parents are uniquely suited to mentalize and understand their children. Steele *et al.* (2007) found that these parents have proven to be, for the most part, resilient and secure in the face of multiple losses and traumatic experiences. Many have been so sensitized by their experiences that they have later chosen to help others at risk.

The children portrayed in this chapter have faced many significant challenges – including difficulties in bonding with others and building up a coherent sense of self – many of which resulted from their unfortunate start in life. Clinicians need to help adoptees and their families learn to tolerate the contradictions, ambiguities and ambivalences that arise while the adopted child matures. If adoptive parents show pride in their family, their children will internalize pride, rather than shame or pain, about being adopted, and the parents in turn will feel pride in the bonds they have nurtured (Pivnick, 2010).

Within the safe context of a therapeutic relationship, a family can find ways to understand the convoluted interactions that occur within their family, with regard to all family members. This chapter did not aim to provide a complete analysis of the complex issues involved in mentalizing, trauma or the interactional problems adoptive families may experience. However, it did set out to provide a better understanding of the important themes our team of psychotherapists and family therapists have encountered during our use of MBT. We hope that other therapists might become more attuned to the problems faced by adoptive families and more capable – if not of always getting it 'right' – then at least of asking 'the right questions'.

References

Adèle. (2008). *To make you feel my love*, 19. Audio CD. London: XL Recordings.

Allen, J. G., Fonagy, P., & Bateman, A. W. (2008). *Mentalizing in clinical practice*. Washington, DC: American Psychiatric Association.

Bleiberg, E. (2001). *Treating personality disorders in children and adolescents: A relational approach*. New York: Guilford Press.

Brodzinsky, D., Smith, D., & Henig, R. (1993). *Being adopted*. New York: Anchor Books.

Brodzinsky, D., Smith, D., & Brodzinsky, A. (1998). *Children's adjustment to adoption: Developmental and clinical issues*. London: Sage

Dozier, M., & Rutter, M. (2008). Challenges to the development of attachment relationships faced by young children in foster and adoptive care. In J. Cassidy & P. R. Shaver (Eds.), *Handbook of attachment, theory, research and clinical applications* (pp. 698–717). New York: Guilford Press.

Fonagy, P., Gergely, G., Jurist, E., & Target, M. (2002). *Affect regulation, mentalization, and the development of the self*. New York: Other Press.

Jemerin, J. (2004). Latency and the capacity to reflect on mental states. *Psychoanalytic Study of the Child*, 59, 211–239.

Johnson, D. E. (2000). Medical and developmental sequelae of early childhood institutionalization in international adoptees from Romania and the Russian Federation. In C. Nelson & N. J. Mahwah (Eds.), *The effects of adversity on neurobehavioral development*. Mahwah, NJ: Lawrence Erlbaum Associates, Inc.

Johnson, D. E. (2002). Adoption and the effect on children's development. *Early Human Development*, 68, 39–54.

Klein, M. (1975). *Envy and gratitude, and other works, 1946–1963*. New York: Free Press.

Kreppner, J. M., O'Connor, T. G., & Rutter, M. (2001). Can inattention/overactivity be an institutional deprivation syndrome? *Journal of Abnormal Child Psychology*, 29, 513–528.

Muller, N., & Kate, C. ten (2008). Mentaliseren bevorderende therapie in relaties en gezinnen. *Tijdschrift voor systeemtherapie*, 3, 117–132.

Muller, N., & Bakker, T. (2009). Oog voor de ouders: Diagnostiek van de hechtingsrelatie tussen ouders en kinderen en het mentaliserend vermogen van ouders. *Tijdschrift voor Kinder en Jeugdpsychotherapie*, 3, 65–79.

Nickman, S. (1985). Losses in adoption: The need for dialogue. *Psychoanalytic Study of the Child*, 40, 365–398.

Ochs, E., & Capps, L. (2001). *Living narrative: Creating lives in everyday storytelling*. Cambridge, MA: Harvard University Press.

Oprell, D. (2005). Adoptiegerelateerde thema's in groepspsychotherapie. In T. J. C. Berk, M. El Bansky, E. Gans, T. A. E. Hoytink, G. H. te Lintelo, G. Missia & M. F. Nout van (Eds.), *Handboek groepstherapie*, Houten: Bohn Stafleu van Loghum.

Pivnick, B. A. (2010). Left without a word: Learning rhythms, rhymes, and reasons in adoption. *Psychoanalytic Inquiry*, 30, 3–24.

Quinodoz, D. (1996). An adopted analysand's transference of a 'hole object'. *International Journal of Psychoanalysis*, 77, 323–336.

Schmeets, M. G. J., & Verheugt-Pleiter, J. E. (2005). *Affectregulatie bij kinderen*. Assen: Koninklijke van Gorcum.

Slade, A. (2010). Reflective parenting programs: Theory and development. *Psychoanalytic Inquiry*, 26(4), 640–657.

Steele, M., Henderson, K., Hodges, J., Kaniuk, J., Hillman, S., & Steele, H. (2007). In the best interest of the late-placed child: A report from the attachment representations and adoption outcome study. In L. Mayes, P. Fonagy & M. Target (Eds.), *Developmental science and psychoanalysis: Integration and innovation* (pp. 159–182). London: Karnac.

Van den Dries, L. (2010). Development after international adoption, PhD thesis. Leiden: University of Leiden.

Van den Dries, L., Juffer, F., Van IJzendoorn, M. H., & Bakermans-Kranenburg, M. J. (2009). Fostering security? A meta-analysis of attachment in adopted children. *Children and Youth Services Review*, 31, 410–421.

Verheugt-Pleiter, A. J. E. (Ed.) (2008). *Mentalizing in child therapy: Guidelines for clinical practitioners*. London: Karnac.

Wallin, D. J. (2007). *Attachment in psychotherapy*. New York: Guilford Press.

Winnicott, D. W. (1992). *The child, the family and the outside world*. New York: Guilford Press.

Chapter 7

Self-harm in young people

Is MBT the answer?

Trudie Rossouw

Here. I'll just post my problems:
Sad a lot.
Like being alone.
Hate being near people.
Veryyyy low self esteem.
I don't like talking around people.
Really weird dreams.
I rarely smile. Sometimes I force myself.
Self-harm, cutting. . . yeah. . . started at age 10.
Scared all the time [anxiety. . .].
Always trying to hide my face.
Death thoughts.
Well, I don't know what else, that's mainly it.
I'm 12 by the way.
My mom has threatened to send me to a psychiatrist around 5 times. . .
never happened. . . even though I wanted it to. . .
[she did because she saw cuts on my arms]
Ugh, what to do?! Ahhh. . .

(From an internet blog about cutting and self-injury)

Self-harm is a common yet complex and quite often serious problem faced by young people today, as well as their families, schools, and mental health services. This chapter has four main aims:

- to introduce self-harm and the controversies surrounding this perplexing phenomenon
- to share an understanding of self-harm within a mentalization-based framework
- to describe a mentalization-based treatment model for young people who harm themselves which is currently being tested with a randomized controlled trial (RCT)

- to share some preliminary analyses exploring the differences between young people who harm themselves and those who do not.

Introducing self-harm

Self-harm has been described in the literature in various ways, but mostly it refers to acts of causing harm to oneself, including self-cutting, burning, self-poisoning, overdosing, attempted hanging, jumping from heights or bridges, etc. Self-harm in young people is highly prevalent and is associated with both morbidity and mortality. The estimate for accident and emergency (A&E) presentations as a result of self-harm in young people annually in England and Wales is 25,000 (Hawton *et al.*, 2000). A national British survey revealed that almost 5 per cent of males and 8 per cent of females aged between 13 and 15 years reported trying to harm, hurt or kill themselves in the previous week (Meltzer *et al.*, 2001). In a large community study in seven EU countries where over 30,000 15- to 16-year-old young people were surveyed, it was found that one in ten females harmed themselves in the previous year (Madge *et al.*, 2008). A community study in Sweden found that 40 per cent of 14 year olds who were questioned engaged in a form of self-harm prior to the interview (Bjärehed & Lundh, 2008). Similarly, a study of 1036 young people in the western part of the USA demonstrated rates of self-cutting that ranged from 26 per cent to 37 per cent (Yates *et al.*, 2008).

Self-harm may or may not express an intention to die. Although distinctive differences between non-suicidal and suicidal self-harming groups of young people have been identified (Jacobson *et al.*, 2008), there is often a great overlap between non-suicidal and suicidal self-harm (Brown, *et al.*, 2002; Nock *et al.*, 2006). For instance, self-harm is the single greatest predictor of completed suicide (Gunnell & Frankel, 1994), with 40–50 per cent of people who die by suicide having a prior history of self-harm (Hawton *et al.*, 2003). In 2002, there were an estimated 877,000 suicides in the world, of which approximately 200,000 were committed by adolescents and young adults (Barker, 2000; Mann *et al.*, 2005).

Increased rates of self-harm have been associated with a range of demographic, family and other factors, including female gender, family conflict, critical parenting, alienation from parents, parental mental health problems, history of physical and sexual abuse, etc. (for a review of the literature, see Evans *et al.*, 2004; Nock *et al.*, 2006). Self-harm has been found in young people with depression (Haavisto *et al.*, 2004), anxiety (Favazza, 1998) and ruminative/negative thinking (Bjärehed & Lundh, 2008). It has also been suggested that self-harm may be a way of decreasing negative mental states such as self-blame, rumination and helplessness (Mikolajczak *et al.*, 2009). Other reasons given for non-suicidal self-injury include attempts at resisting thoughts of suicide, a way to express self-anger or disgust, efforts to escape times of dissociation, wishes to influence others, or a wish to seek help from others (Klonsky & Muehlenkamp, 2007; Walsh, 2007).

Whether or not self-harm is indicative of underlying personality pathology, and in particular borderline personality disorder (BPD), has been a topic of great controversy. On the one hand, several studies have established a strong link between personality disturbance and self-harm. For instance, among adolescents who engaged in both non-suicidal and suicidal self-harm, rates of BPD were found to be elevated, whereas major depression and post traumatic stress disorder (PTSD) were predictive of membership in the suicidal group (Jacobson *et al.*, 2008). However, BPD has been also found to be the personal disorder most highly correlated with suicide attempts in a clinical sample of adolescents (Westen *et al.*, 2003). From a longitudinal perspective, Levy (2005) found that one-third of individuals diagnosed with BPD engaged in self-harm before age 12, and likewise it has been found retrospectively that self-harm, when present in childhood and adolescence, is an early risk indicator for BPD in adulthood (Zanarini *et al.*, 2006).

On the other hand, it has been pointed out that a significant percentage of people who engage in self-harm during adolescence will not develop BPD in adulthood (Siever *et al.*, 2002). In other studies, young people engaging in both suicidal and non-suicidal self-harm were more likely to qualify for a wide range of Axis I rather than Axis II disorders (Nock *et al.*, 2006; Portzky *et al.*, 2008).

Making sense of self-harm: a mentalization-based framework

As has been described in some detail in the first chapter, mentalization is a skill that develops in the context of an attachment relationship. At birth human infants are unable to regulate their emotions themselves (Fonagy, 2000). To acquire this capacity the infant requires the caregiver to accurately understand and respond to the moment-to-moment changes in the infant's emotional state (Fonagy, 2000). This is thought to be achieved through the caregiver mirroring back to the baby their emotional experience in a marked way, which labels it and communicates that it is controllable. The markedness of the mirroring signals that it is symbolic of the baby's, not the mother's own emotional state, and forms what has been termed a 'secondary representation' of the experience in the baby's mind (Bateman & Fonagy, 2004). This gradually forms the 'core self' in the baby (Fonagy, 2000). The core self therefore is a representation based on the caregiver's understanding of the infant's feelings as well as the caregiver's perception of the infant as an intentional being. This leads to an inner representation in the infant of himself/herself as an intentional/agentive being and this is thought to generalize to the representation of others leading to the development of a mentalizing model of the world (Fonagy, 2000), which helps the child to perceive the relational world as meaningful and predictable and to respond to the complexities of social reality with resilience (Fonagy, 2000).

When the caregiver's representations of the infant are based on misattuned attributions, the infant will internalize inaccurate representations of him or herself and hence the secondary representation in the infant's mind will be alien to the authentic mental state and intentionality of the infant. This alien representation, however, becomes part of the inner self concept and has been labelled the 'alien self' by Fonagy (2000). Repeated experiences of this kind will finally lead to a situation where the infant or young child's mind is dominated by the alien self. The inner experience of the alien self is akin to the experience of an inner tormentor – it is the constant experience of inner criticism, self hatred, lack of internal validation and expectation of failure. The self is hated and through the projected lens of the alien self the external world can be perceived as potentially hostile, humiliating and attacking.

In an internal state dominated by the alien self where the inner representations are incongruent with one's experiences, representations of others will be similarly inaccurate and will therefore lead to the experience that the relational world does not make sense and neither is it predictable or manageable. In this way the alien self may hinder the development of mentalization.

Within this perspective, self-harm is understood as both symptomatic of a deficit in the capacity to mentalize (Bateman & Fonagy, 2004), and as an attempt to liberate the self from the alien self (Fonagy *et al.*, 2002). Thus, self-harm represents a concrete way of managing strong emotions in the context of a breakdown in the ability to attend to mental states in the self and others. In this non-mentalizing mode, 'parts of the body may be considered equivalent to specific mental states and can thus be literally physically removed' (Bateman & Fonagy, 2006: 27). What follows is an example demonstrating how the alien self of a girl called Sally expresses itself in the presence of non-mentalizing cycles:

Sally starts to feel anxious because she had a bad day at school and felt bullied by the other children. When she feels anxious she starts to believe that there is something wrong with her body, such as that she might be having a heart attack. She then feels terrified that she may die.

Action: She rushes to her mother and insists on being taken to hospital.
Impact: Her mother feels irritated by this demand as she has learnt over time that there is nothing physically wrong with Sally, and that no matter how many times she and the doctor have told this to Sally, she does not listen. Her mother thinks Sally is just attention seeking.

Action: Sally's mother tells her to go away and that she is imagining it.
Impact: This makes Sally feel that her mother was not listening to her and this makes her furious.
Action: Sally goes to her room and starts throwing things out of the window.
Impact: Sally's mother gets angry and frightened that the situation is going to get out of hand.
Action: She tells Sally to go into the garden and locks her out of the house.
Impact: Sally feels that her mother does not love her and therefore feels desperate. She feels horrible, bad and unlovable and starts to panic.
Action: Sally starts throwing bricks at the window to be let in.
Impact: Now Sally's mother starts to feel frightened of her. She is frightened Sally will break a window and hurt her two other children; she feels helpless and unable to know what to do. She starts to panic and finally calls the police. At this stage she feels incompetent as a parent, helpless and frightened.

At the crescendo moment of such an escalating cycle both parties feel like victims. Not only do both parties feel attacked by the other, but both experience terribly bad feelings about themselves. They feel mean, incompetent, unlovable, etc. If we as clinicians intervene in a situation where the alien self is activated, it is extremely important to be aware of the proneness for people to feel blamed or attacked under such circumstances.

The golden rule is to form an empathic alliance with the experience of people in this state, acknowledging how hard it is to feel that whatever you try fails and that you are to blame for this. In that way we make empathic contact with the authentic self, which in turn creates an experience of safety in the alliance and a reprieve from the onslaught of the alien self. This alliance will create the space for reflection, which will set the stage for efforts to mentalize where things went wrong. Once mentalization is restored, the influence of the alien self will be reduced.

Mentalization-based treatment for adolescents (MBT-A)

MBT-A is a modified version of the adult MBT treatment developed by Bateman and Fonagy (2006). It is a structured and manualized treatment model which consists of once weekly individual MBT treatment for the young person combined with monthly or twice monthly mentalization-based therapy for families (MBT-F). All therapists providing the treatment are child and adolescent mental health services (CAMHS) professionals who underwent additional training in the model.

The primary aim of MBT-A is to help young people and their families improve their awareness of their own mental states and the mental states of others through the enhancement of mentalization capacity. The emphasis is on improving their understanding of mental states and processes that drive behaviour and relational patterns, as opposed to exploring the unconscious content driving these states or applying behaviourally derived management strategies to specific behavioural symptoms of distress.

The underlying concept fundamental to practising MBT is that behaviour difficulties and/or escalating family conflict regularly result from a failure in mentalization. Central to the understanding of these processes is the impact of mentalization failure on emotional regulation. MBT proposes that failure in mentalization can instigate affect dysregulation within an individual which in turn produces further mentalization failure. Such emotional dysregulation in one individual rarely exists in a bubble of isolation from which all others are spared. Instead, the mounting dysregulation and the mentalization failure migrate into the individual's interpersonal world where many relationships fall prey to escalating interpersonal misunderstanding and conflict. Furthermore, the spread of mentalization failure often culminates in some form of concrete acts or 'acting out' behaviours exhibited by the individuals involved – be it through self-harm, physical violence, slamming doors, breaking things, taking drugs, or running away. It is because of this process that the emphasis of MBT is not on managing the symptomatic, overt behaviours, but rather on understanding the multitude of ways in which mentalization has broken down, and the ways in which this affects people within an individual's social system.

Key elements of this structure include: a theoretically coherent treatment approach; a mentalizing clinical team; and consistent application of the approach over time. In dealing with young people and their families where the currency of communication and managing of emotions has become action and acting out behaviour, the therapist may be invited, and expected, to do some form of action in order to intervene. Many of us will be familiar with how easy it is to give a knee jerk response, usually involving some form of action, in order to manage the immediate anxiety or provocation of particular forms of acting out behaviour. As described above, highly aroused states in an individual easily induce aroused states in those around them. The therapist and the treatment team are not immune to this experience, and along with others they will experience at these times increased emotional arousal and therefore challenges facing their ability to mentalize. It is for this reason that a mentalizing team that is offering regular supervision without sitting in the heat of the arousal can help the therapist refrain from acting impulsively in response to emotionally charged interactions, and restore their own mentalizing abilities so that an understanding of these highly arousing interactions can start to develop.

MBT-A consists of the assessment phase and three treatment phases: the initial treatment phase, the middle phase and the final phase. The *assessment phase* lasts for about two sessions and its aim is to form a psychological formulation of the young person's difficulties. Some Axis I disorders may need treatment in their own right with medication. It is also important to get an idea of the young person's cognitive abilities as difficulties in this area may interfere with the ability to mentalize. During the assessment we also try to assess the young person's and their family's ability to mentalize, and we try to establish which contexts may trigger the collapse of mentalization. In some cases, concern over the mental health of one of the parents may be highlighted and in those cases the parent may require additional help for themselves from adult services.

The *initial treatment phase* starts with the formulation meeting, in which the young person is presented with a written formulation (an example is available from the author on request). In the family meeting the formulation is not presented in a written format, but forms the basis of a discussion. The aim of the formulation is to explain the current difficulties in mentalizing and relational terms. Its aim is also to present to the young people and their families an image of themselves that will make them feel understood. It should help them too see themselves objectively, and also to become aware of the subjective experience of others. The formulation also provides a springboard for outlining a treatment pathway that could assist the young person and their family to gain a sense of control. The family formulation refers to family members' understanding of one another as well as how they feel affected by each other. The formulation is discussed and altered depending on the outcome of the meeting with the young person. The formulation also includes a crisis plan and lastly at the end of the formulation meeting the contract is discussed. This is a discussion about the practicalities of the treatment, the duration, the frequency of sessions and some expected forms of behaviour from all parties, such as specifying the required commitment to the work and agreeing not to use violence or drugs.

After the formulation meeting with the family the psychoeducation meeting follows. In some settings it has been found that it is easier for this to be done in larger groups of families. The aim of psychoeducation is to help families take on board the principle that behaviour has meaning, that feelings arise in a relational context and that people have a powerful emotional impact on one another. The format of the psychoeducation varies. In some settings it is an informal discussion with the family by using the examples from their everyday life and in the multi-family group it involves more direct input and the use of discussion, games, role plays and video material.

The aim of the *middle phase* is to enhance mentalization in the young person and their family, which will include the ability to become more aware of mental states in others. The aim here is to turn around non-mentalizing and coercive ways of interacting into mentalizing ways where there is more understanding of one another, trust and clearer communications, and where helplessness and passivity are turned around into a sense of mastery. Helping the young person and the family gain better impulse control is another aim of this phase, as the lack of impulse control continuously undermines the development of mentalizing abilities. This facilitates the introduction of specific interventions to manage suicidal, parasuicidal, and other harmful or impulsive behaviours such as substance abuse, bingeing and purging, fits of rage, or threatening behaviour (Bleiberg *et al.*, 2012).

The *final phase* involves consolidating the gains made in therapy, preparing the young person and their family for independence and helping the young person towards greater responsibility.

In our trial, MBT-A is a treatment programme for one year whereas treatment as usual can be of any duration. The results will be disseminated in future publications upon completion of the trial.

Below is an example of MBT-A with a 15-year-old young man, John, who was referred to our service with a history of cutting himself, taking overdoses and having great difficulty in managing relations at school. He also has a strong history of violent outbursts and impulsive behaviour including one incident in which he was reprimanded by the police for attacking another young man.

John grew up with his mother and two half siblings from different fathers. His mother has a past history of drug abuse. The young man experienced life as unpredictable. He grew up surrounded by volatile relationships and consistently experienced inconsistent boundaries. This upbringing meant he had very limited ability to manage his own feelings and hence frequently fell back on concrete ways of trying to reassure himself of his safety and of managing his feelings. This extract below from one of his sessions illustrates both his concrete mentalizing style and the therapist's attempts to help him mentalize his feelings.

John: I broke up with Michelle. You remember I wanted to see her last Friday and she said she was busy. Later I found out that she was only busy for one hour and I could have seen her. So Saturday I thought I am not having it, I may as well end it with her rather than wait around for her. I sent her a text and said, 'If you do not call by 5 o'clock it is over.' She texted straight back saying 'I am sorry but I am a happy person and you are always moaning and it brings me down.' So I thought: 'OK, whatever', and just left it.

Therapist: Gosh, what did that make you feel?

John: I felt nothing. I just don't understand, I was always happy when I was with her. I don't see how she could say I am always moaning. The only thing I moaned about was that she just never answered her phone. Any boyfriend would want that, isn't it?

Therapist: So when she did not answer her phone, what did you feel?

John: It felt as if she did not care. Jenny always answered her phone and that is how I knew she cared.

Therapist: And when you felt she did not care, what did you do?

John: I would phone her non-stop and I would text and leave messages. It is not right to ignore me like this. I sometimes called her 20 times and she would ignore me. I then think she's met someone else. And I sort of saw it coming, so Friday evening when I went dancing I flirted with people and then I met this new girl. So I thought I'd like to take her out, so I pretended to be drunk and then said to her that I would like to take her out. I thought if I pretend to be drunk and if she says no, then I will just say the next day that I was drunk and that I do not remember anything. Then I won't have to feel embarrassed. But she did not do that, she said she'd like to go out with me. So Saturday when I dumped Michelle I already had the other one lined up, so I did not really care about Michelle anymore. So now life has moved on and this weekend I will go out with her for the first time. And this week I felt really happy. This girl is really special. We have so much in common, she is pretty. . .

Therapist: Can I just slow things down a bit to try and catch up?

John: Yes, it is a bit fast, isn't it? I always do that, I always have one in reserve. The minute I see trouble coming I get one in reserve.

Therapist: It seems to me all of this action about phoning her so many times and getting another girl in reserve are all ways in which you try and manage a terribly anxious feeling inside you.

John: Yes but now I don't feel it, because the new girl answers her phone all the time, just like Jenny did, so it helps me.

Therapist: So when Michelle did not answer her phone, what did you feel?

John: I felt anxious that she was seeing another guy and then I phoned again and again.

Therapist: If I think someone I like is seeing someone else, it would make me feel angry.

John: Yes I felt I could smash my phone up. I wanted to break her door down.

Therapist: So part of phoning her so many times was also an angry thing?

John: Yes, I suppose it is a bit smothering, maybe that is why she said I was moaning. But any guy will be upset if he is ignored. . .

In a further example of concrete mentalizing Darren, a 16-year-old man came to his outpatient session stating that he was upset about his girlfriend being unfaithful to him and that he was going to 'dump' her after the session. The evidence of her unfaithfulness, he told me, was in a text he received from her. He then read the text to me and it said something about her wish to be with him and that she was going to break it off with her previous boyfriend. She ended the text with the sentence 'I will tell him that.' I did not understand what was upsetting to him about the text, so asked for clarification. He explained that if she had said 'I will tell him that when I see him next', it would mean she was going to see him in the future, but instead her saying 'I will tell him that' meant she was with him when she sent the text. In Darren's mind if his girlfriend was with her ex-boyfriend, then she was unfaithful to him. In his rage, and driven by his impulsivity, he wanted to send her an immediate text to tell her never to contact him again. With careful work I stopped him from acting out, slowed him down and helped him to see his distortion and how in his distortion he missed the true message of the text, which was about her love for him. Only after he calmed down, and after he was less impulsive and more in touch with her as a person with feelings towards him, could we explore his deep fear that she would leave him.

Is there evidence for the alien self?

In order to explore the distinguishing differences between young people who harm themselves and those who do not, our research team conducted a cross-sectional study comparing a self-harming group (n=80) against two non-self-harming control groups: a non-clinical school group (n=34) and a non-self-harming clinical group of young people presenting to CAMHS with other difficulties (n=30).

The study was conducted in the North East London Foundation Trust, covering a population of one million people. All young people were between 12 and 17 years old. Those who presented to CAMHS services meeting criteria for either the self-harming or the non-self-harming control group were invited to participate in the study. The school group was recruited by targeting schools in the same areas as the self-harm group and asking young people of the same age to volunteer to participate in the research. Young people with moderate to severe learning disability (LD), autism spectrum disorder (ASD), psychosis or eating disorder without additional self-harm were excluded from the study.

The groups were assessed in terms of risk taking behaviour, personality features, mood, attachment styles, dissociation and mentalization. (A list of the measures used is available from the author on request.) Analysis of the data showed that young people in the self-harm group were significantly more depressed, had significantly higher levels of dissociation, childhood abuse and substance misuse proneness than both the school and the clinical control group ($p<.001$). There was no significant difference in terms of anxiety.

In terms of personality style, the self-harm group displayed significantly higher borderline traits ($p<.001$) and young people in the self-harm group were more likely to meet full criteria for BPD diagnosis compared to those in the other two groups. In addition, the self-harming group was significantly more introversive/avoidant ($p<.001$) and self-demeaning ($p<.001$)

than the control groups. In light of the abusive experiences most of them have experienced, the avoidant trait could be then understood as a self preservative consequence of the abuse.

Could the avoidant trait also be seen as possibly indicative of the alien self? A common manifestation of the alien self is the externalization of it, i.e. the expectation to be attacked and humiliated. If someone is filled with such anxieties, then it would make sense that they are very cautious of the external world and hence become avoidant. Could the higher scores on self-demeaning traits also be understood as evidence of the alien self? As the alien self has been described like an internal tormentor, young people driven by such an internal constellation are likely to perceive themselves in negative terms, undermine themselves and present themselves in a negative light to others, which are elements of the self-demeaning trait.

Interestingly, the control groups were significantly more dramatizing (p<.001), submissive (p<.001 between the self-harm groups and schools, and p<.05 between the self-harm and the clinical control), egotistic and conforming (p<.001) than the self-harm group. These traits could be understood as indicative of someone's perception that they can elicit help from those around them, in other words, a more benign perception of the world around them. This could in turn be seen as evidence of the absence of an alien self, which may act as a protective factor in these groups. Because if young people are able to elicit help from those around them at times of struggle, they will be better able to get help with affect regulation and hence will be more likely to retain their capacity for mentalization. This will also buffer them against experiences of isolation and loneliness. The two control groups were also more egotistic which could be seen as indicative of them having higher self regard than the self-harm group, which again could be interpreted possibly as evidence of the absence of an alien self.

Along similar lines, one of the mentalizing scales demonstrated that the school group was significantly better at mentalizing than the self-harm group (p<.01). However, other mentalizing scales did not detect any differences between the three groups, and this may have to do with challenges related to measuring context-specific, 'on-line' mentalization, which are discussed in Chapter 3.

In terms of attachment, the self-harm group appeared significantly more anxious (p<.01) and avoidant (p<.01) compared to the other groups. Moreover, feelings of alienation from parents were significantly higher in the self-harm group than in the control groups (p<.001), but interestingly the three groups did not differ in their feelings of alienation from peers. Conversely, communication with parents was higher in the control groups than in the self-harm group (p<.001 for the contrast between the self-harm and the school group). These findings are in line with a large body of evidence suggesting an important link between specific attachment organizations and self-harm in adolescence.

Conclusion

Self-harm is a serious mental health problem with prevalence rates that remain high and are rising among young people in the western world. The goal of this chapter was to present a theoretical, mentalization-based formulation of self-harm in young people, focusing largely on the concept of the alien self, and the impairment of mentalization in the context of insecure attachment. Based on the very promising results of studies looking at MBT for adults with BPD (Bateman & Fonagy, 1999, 2009) we applied the principles of MBT in a treatment programme for young people who present with self-harm. This chapter offered clinical examples of mentalization failures and described attempts at restoring mentalization within an MBT-A session. This chapter also presented the results from our cross-sectional study comparing a self-harming group of young people with a clinical and a community control group. Our findings suggest that the profile of young people who self-harm is consistent with a mentalization-based understanding of self-harm. The RCT will be completed in the near future and evidence about the efficacy of MBT-A will become available and will hopefully provide a framework for effective intervention and prevention.

References

Barker, G. (2000). What about boys: A literature review in the health and development of adolescent boys. Geneva: WHO Department of Child and Adolescent Health and Development.

Bateman, A., & Fonagy, P. (1999). The effectiveness of partial hospitalization in the treatment of borderline personality disorder – a randomized controlled trial. *American Journal of Psychiatry*, 156, 1563–1569.

Bateman, A., & Fonagy, P. (2004). *Psychotherapy for borderline personality disorder: Mentalization-based treatment*. Oxford: Oxford University Press.

Bateman, A., & Fonagy, P. (2006). *Mentalization-based treatment for borderline personality disorder: A practical guide*. Oxford: Oxford University Press.

Bateman, A., & Fonagy, P. (2009). Randomised control trial of outpatient treatment versus clinical management for borderline personality disorder. *American Journal of Psychology*, 166(12), 1355–1364.

Bjärehed, J., & Lundh, L. (2008). Deliberate self-harm in 14-year-old adolescents: How frequent is it, and how is it associated with psychopathology, relationship variables, and styles of emotional regulation? *Cognitive Behaviour Therapy*, 37(1), 26–37.

Bleiberg, E., Rossouw, T., & Fonagy, P. (2012). Adolescent breakdown and emerging personality disorder. In A.W. Bateman & P. Fonagy (Eds.), *Handbook of mentalizing in mental health practice* (pp. 463–509). Washington, DC: American Psychiatric Publishing.

Brown, M. Z., Comtois, K. A., & Linehan, M. M. (2002). Reasons for suicide attempts and nonsuicidal self-injury in women with borderline personality disorder. *Journal of Abnormal Psychology*, 111, 198–202.

Evans, E., Hawton, K., & Rodham, K. (2004). Factors associated with suicidal phenomena in adolescents: A systematic review of population-based studies. *Clinical Psychology Review*, 24, 957–979.

Favazza, A. R. (1998). The coming of age of self-mutilation. *Journal of Nervous & Mental Disease*, 186(5), 259–268.

Fonagy, P. (2000). Attachment and borderline personality disorder. *Journal of the American Psychoanalytic Association*, 48, 1129–1146.

Fonagy, P., Gergely, G., Jurist, E., & Target, M. (2002). *Affect regulation, mentalization and the development of the self.* New York: Other Press.

Gunnell, D., & Frankel, S. (1994). Prevention of suicide: Aspirations and evidence. *British Medical Journal*, 308, 1227–1233.

Haavisto, A., Sourander, A., Multimaki, P., Parkkola, K., Santalahti, P., Helenius, H., *et al.* (2004). Factors associated with depressive symptoms among 18-year-old boys: A prospective 10-year follow-up study. *Journal of Affective Disorders*, 83(2–3), 143–154.

Hawton, K., Fagg, J., Simkin, S., Bale, E., & Bond, A. (2000). Deliberate self-harm in adolescents in Oxford, 1985–1995. *Journal of Adolescence*, 23(1), 47–55.

Hawton, K., Hall, S., Simkin, S., Bale, E., Bond, A., Codd, S., & Stewart, A. (2003). Deliberate self-harm in adolescents: A study of characteristics and trends in Oxford, 1990–2000. *Journal of Child Psychology and Psychiatry and Allied Disciplines*, 44, 1191–1198.

Jacobson, C., Muehlenkamp, M., Miller, A. L., & Turner, B. J. (2008). Psychiatric impairment among adolescents engaging in different types of deliberate self-harm. *Journal of Clinical Child and Adolescent Psychology*, 37(2), 363–375.

Klonsky, E. D., & Muehlenkamp, J. J. (2007). Self-injury: A research review for the practitioner. *Journal of Clinical Psychology*, 63, 1045–1056.

Levy, K. N. (2005). The implications of attachment theory and research for understanding borderline personality disorder. *Development and Psychopathology*, 17(4), 959–986.

Madge, N., Hewitt, A., Howton, K., de Wilde, E. J., Corcoran, P., Fekete, S., *et al.* (2008). Deliberate self-harm within an international community sample of young people: Comparative findings from the Child and Adolescent Self-harm in Europe (CASE) study. *Journal of Child Psychology and Psychiatry*, 49(6), 667–677.

Mann, J. J., Apter, A., Bertolote, J., Beautrais, A., Currier, D., Haas, A., *et al.* (2005). Suicide prevention strategies: A systematic review. *Journal of American Medical Association*, 294, 2064–2074.

Meltzer, H., Harrington, R., Goodman, R., & Jenkins, R. (2001). *Children and adolescents who try to kill themselves.* London: Office for National Statistics.

Mikolajczak, M., Petrides, K., & Hurry, J. (2009). Adolescents choosing self-harm as an emotion regulation strategy: The protective role of trait emotional intelligence. *British Journal of Clinical Psychology*, 48, 181–193.

Nock, M., Joiner, T. E., Gordon, K. H., Lloyd-Richardson, E., & Prinstein, M. J. (2006). Non-suicidal self-injury among adolescents: Diagnostic correlates and relation to suicide attempts. *Psychiatry Research*, 144, 65–72.

Portzky, G., de Wilde, E. J., & van Heeringen, K. (2008). Deliberate self-harm in young people: Differences in prevalence and risk factors between the Netherlands and Belgium. *European Child Adolescent Psychiatry*, 17, 179–186.

Siever, L. J., Torgersen, S., Gunderson, J. G., Livesley, W. J., & Kendler, K. S. (2002). The borderline diagnosis III: Identifying endophenotypes for genetic studies. *Biological Psychiatry*, 51, 964–968.

Walsh, B. (2007). Clinical assessment of self-injury: A practical guide. *Journal of Clinical Psychology*, 63, 1057–1068.

Westen, D., Shedler, J., Durrett, C., Glass, S., & Martens, A. (2003). Personality diagnoses in adolescence: DSM-IV Axis II diagnoses and an empirically derived alternative. *American Journal of Psychiatry*, 160, 952–966.

Yates, T. M., Tracy, A. J., & Luthar, S. S. (2008). Nonsuicidal self-injury among 'privileged' youths: Longitudinal and cross-sectional approaches to developmental process. *Journal of Consulting Clinical Psychology*, 76, 52–62.

Zanarini, M. C., Frankenburg, F. R., Ridolfi, M. E., Jager-Hyman, S., Hennen, J., & Gunderson, J. G. (2006). Reported childhood onset of self-mutilation among borderline patients. *Journal of Personality Disorders*, 20(1), 9–15.

Part III

Community-based interventions

Chapter 8

Thinking and feeling in the context of chronic illness

A mentalization-based group intervention with adolescents

Norka T. Malberg

Introduction

In 1965, Thesi Bergmann in collaboration with Anna Freud wrote a book about working with children in a hospital setting. When describing what they thought would be needed for such work, they wrote:

> Technique will have to be flexible, that is, applicable to disturbances which range from the surface to the depth. Since therapy is carried out within the hospital setting, it has to involve not only the parents of the patient but equally the nursing and medical staff. Since the approach ranges from the human to the scientific and covers every aspect of the child's life, an orientation in these various fields will be essential for the worker, so will observational skill and a thorough grounding in the essentials of a developmental child psychology.
>
> (Bergmann & Freud, 1965: 151)

The tradition of exploring effective ways of serving the mental health needs of young people in hospital represents one of the many contributions made by Anna Freud to the field of child and adolescent psychotherapy (A. Freud, 1952). The early work of Thesi Bergmann and Anna Freud, and later the systematic research on psychoanalytic treatment in hospitals carried out by Fonagy and Moran (1990), invited and challenged psychotherapists working within the walls of the paediatric unit in two ways: not only to explore the impact of somatic illness on the internal development and functioning of the child, but also to observe and integrate the study of the different external social systems supporting the child during the traumatic experience of illness into their understanding and models of treatment. Such work has had a profound influence on the work of psychodynamic child psychotherapists working in hospital settings (Ramsden, 1999).

This chapter will illustrate how the application of vital components of the psychoanalytic method and theory can prove beneficial in the process of fostering a secure and contained environment where young chronically ill adolescents can safely explore the subjective meaning of the experience of illness. This goal was achieved by the integration of classical psychoanalytic concepts, like the analysis of defence, with constructs from attachment theory and the social cognitive school of thought, with its interest in topics such as perspective taking and the capacity to mentalize. The following pages describe the context and development of a clinical application of these ideas on a paediatric haemodialysis unit in the UK serving eight adolescent patients (aged 12 to 17) experiencing end stage renal disease (ESRD). The intervention sought to activate the attachment system of these adolescents with the purpose of influencing positively their capacity to think about the impact of their feelings on their adherence to the medical regime. Furthermore, I underline the vital role of a secondary goal: that of promoting mentalizing within the relational systems surrounding the chronically ill young person. In Thesi Bergmann's words, I hope to illustrate the value of 'mental first aid' when provided in an integrative manner.

The experience of paediatric end stage renal disease

One of the biggest challenges of being part of the hospital system is learning to understand the illness and the language that parents, young people and medical staff share in common, what one of our patients called 'sick talk', i.e. the language regarding medical procedures and conditions. For this reason, I will begin by providing a brief review of what constitutes paediatric kidney disease and the reality of its treatment in order to offer the reader a framework and a window into the experience of the young person suffering from end stage renal disease (ESRD).

Medical facts

The risk of kidney failure increases significantly with age, with children under the age of 19 presenting an annual rate of only one or two cases in every 100,000 (NKUDIC, 2010). However, contemporary medical advances have increased the likelihood of children surviving with chronic conditions, thereby increasing the numbers of children and adolescents living with one or more chronic conditions. As a result, there has been an increasing need to explore creative and innovative ways of serving the psychosocial needs of such children. This is especially relevant when their eligibility for and success of transplantation are so closely related to their capacity to adhere to the medical regime.

The kidneys are responsible for vital functions in our bodies. When blood flows through the kidneys, waste products and extra water are removed from the blood and sent to the bladder as urine. The kidneys also regulate blood pressure, balance chemicals like sodium and potassium, and make hormones to help bones grow and keep the blood healthy by making new red blood cells. The causes of chronic renal failure include anatomic (birth defects, hereditary disease), immunologic (caused by lupus or diabetes) and miscellaneous factors or conditions (e.g. glomerular disease) which may lead to irreversible abnormalities of kidney function.

A child whose kidneys have failed completely must receive treatment to replace the work the kidneys do. The two types of treatment are dialysis and transplantation. The two main types of dialysis are peritoneal dialysis and haemodialysis. Peritoneal dialysis can be done at home; it involves using the lining of the child's abdominal cavity, the peritoneum, as a filter. A catheter placed in the child's belly is used to pour a solution containing dextrose (a sugar) into the abdominal cavity. While the solution is there, it pulls water and extra fluid from the blood. Later, the solution is drained from the belly, along with the wastes and extra fluid. The cavity is then refilled and the cleaning process continues (NKUDIC, 2010). This method can be used without the supervision of medical personnel. However, the young person and his family tend to receive training before they are allowed to perform this treatment at home. Families often complain of the process being difficult and at times interfering with social activities of the families and the young person.

The other method of dialysis is haemodialysis. This method uses a machine that carries the child's blood through a tube to a dialyzer, a canister that contains thousands of fibres that filter out the wastes and extra fluid. The cleaned blood is then returned to the child through a different tube. This process is generally carried out in the hospital and generally takes place three times a week for about three to four hours each time. Many young people in the haemodialysis unit have experienced failed transplants. Others are asked to attend the unit as their home environment would not sustain the strain of peritoneal dialysis or because they have other accompanying illnesses which require closer medical supervision.

Transplantation provides the closest thing to a cure for kidney failure. There are two types of transplants: from a living donor (in many instances family members but not necessarily so) or from a deceased donor. After transplantation the young person must take medications to keep the body's immune system from rejecting the new organ. These medications help the organ to stay healthy but make the young person more vulnerable to infections.

Perhaps the most devastating physical consequence of chronic renal disease in children is the development of bone disease with associated deformities. These may prevent adequate ambulation and impair growth and sexual development with its profound effects on psychosocial adaptation. Young people undergoing haemodialysis have daily dietary restrictions determined by their individual conditions which often include restricted liquid and caloric intake. All these medical restrictions and procedures tend to have a negative impact on the young people's psychosocial development and functioning.

Psychosocial impact of ESRD and other chronic illnesses on adolescents

The problems of psychosocial adjustment to end stage renal disease (ESRD) during childhood and adolescence have received considerable research attention. A number of studies have identified the effects of renal failure on growth and physical appearance as a major concern for children in dialysis (Reynolds *et al.*, 1986). Increased levels of anxiety, low self-esteem and behavioural disturbance have also been reported (Henning *et al.*, 1988). The time taken up by dialysis and associated hospital visits and admissions may cause considerable disruption to normal social activity and school attendance (Garralda *et al.*, 1988) and educational under-functioning is therefore common (Poursanidou *et al.*, 2003). Additional stress may also arise from the medical procedures carried out during treatment and repeated hospitalizations (Garralda *et al.*, 1988).

Studies have also demonstrated the effects that a child's ESRD and dialysis treatment may have on other family members. Parental relationship problems, high levels of anxiety, depression and psychosomatic problems in parents, and family burnout have all been noted (Brownbridge & Fielding, 1994). The process of haemodialysis can be extremely frustrating and time-consuming for the child and his family as it significantly affects school attendance and leisure time. Furthermore, it often disrupts parents' work obligations as well as siblings' social activities. It is not uncommon to find older siblings being used as escorts, particularly during weekend sessions. As a result, the process of haemodialysis presents the young person and his environment with considerable stressors.

Recently, there has been a focus in the literature on the promotion of interventions that foster the exploration of specific factors such as culture and spirituality and their impact on the individual meaning of the illness. For instance, Soliday *et al.* (2000) highlight the need for clinicians to promote children's well-being by focusing on strengths identified by parents such as a sense of humour, spirit, love of life and pro-social behaviour. Clay *et al.* (2002) underlined the importance of exploring how culture influences health care beliefs, practices, health care utilization and adherence. For example, cultural beliefs about the causes and remedies for illness can influence attitudes towards medical regimes. In this way, incongruence between such beliefs and assumptions can result in a disengagement from the medical team and poor adherence to treatment.

Non-adherence is common in patients undergoing chronic haemodialysis (Curtin *et al.*, 1999; Leggat *et al.*, 1998; Swartz, 1998). Depending on the definition used, as many as 86 per cent of dialysis patients may be considered non-adherent with one or more aspects of their treatment but the median is closer to 50 per cent. In a study of children and adolescents (Brownbridge & Fielding, 1994), low adherence with dialysis treatment (assessed by self report, weight gain, blood pressure and serum potassium and blood urea levels) correlated with poor adjustment to dialysis, anxiety and depression, low socioeconomic status and poor family structure. These findings are similar to those reported in studies of adult dialysis patients. For the chronically ill adolescent, attitudes and therapeutic motivation, the personal meaning and significance of the illness and treatment are the most important factors affecting compliance (Kyngas *et al.*, 2000). Anderson *et al.* (1997) point to the importance of the patients' feeling that they achieve valuable personal goals as a result of good adherence.

Group modalities working with chronically ill adolescents

Adolescents spend most of their daytime hours in school or leisure settings with friends. The adolescent in haemodialysis spends 12 hours a week with peers in three times weekly sessions at the unit. As a result, there seems to be the assumption amongst medical personnel that attending the haemodialysis unit will provide the young person with a support network of peers who understand the challenges and limitations of being a young person suffering from ESRD. However, this assumption has been shown to be incorrect. For example, when Garralda *et al.* (1988) compared the psychiatric adjustment in children with chronic renal insufficiency (CRI), haemodialysis patients and healthy children, they reported a trend towards higher internalizing symptoms (anxiety, worrying, depressive symptoms) for children in both illness groups, indicating that young people in the haemodialysis category are as vulnerable as those in the other clinical group.

During adolescence, close friendships represent a significant source of emotional support and may facilitate adolescents' adjustment to a chronic disease or their ability to cope with a difficult medical treatment. As a result, additional efforts are needed to examine the potential positive influences that friends/close peers may have on the adolescent's disease management and adaptative health behaviours (Burroughs *et al.*, 1993). Although individual psychotherapy is the most common format for treatment in clinical settings, nearly half of all child and adolescent clinical treatment outcome studies have assessed the efficacy of treatments provided within a group context (Kazdin & Weisz, 1998). Group treatment may be particularly beneficial to children with medical conditions for two very significant reasons. First, social adjustment is an area of particular vulnerability for young people with chronic illnesses, and peer relationships may affect adaptation to the disease (Haberbeck-Weber & McKee, 1995). Second, groups offer participants opportunities for modelling, problem solving, helping others and relating to peers who share similar circumstances, all of which are more difficult to provide through individual therapy.

A review of group interventions for paediatric chronic conditions carried out by Plante and colleagues (2001) indicated that group interventions have been used with a variety of paediatric populations to increase knowledge of the medical condition, increase adaptation to the illness and reduce physical symptoms. However, the review points out to the fact that there is need for well-controlled studies of emotional support groups as well as psychoeducational ones. The mentalization-based group intervention attempts to fill that gap by developing a model of intervention based on detailed observation and integration of modalities using existing research findings and the application of clinical constructs which have shown to be successful working with this population in the past.

The mentalization-based therapy group model: how and why?

The mentalization-based group model provides a 'relational laboratory' where the chronically ill young person can safely explore his thoughts and feelings about the illness and its impact on his overall development and functioning within the world of relationships. In other words, it allows for the contained exploration of the individual meaning of a traumatic experience, which often impairs the young person's capacity to mentalize his behaviours when confronted with both normative interpersonal conflicts as well as conflicts stemming from the context of illness. A mentalization-based therapy group with chronically ill adolescents (MBTG-A; Malberg *et al.*, 2008) has the following main aims:

- To reactivate the attachment system by focusing on themes that are emotionally, developmentally and culturally relevant to the young person. This includes discussing a range of topics, from exploring the experience of chronic illness to age-related concerns such as difficulties with peers.
- To restore the capacity for thinking about feelings whilst still experiencing the emotional state that often causes the young person to engage in 'non-mentalizing relational exchanges'.
- To identify maladaptive defensive strategies and to provide new ego-strengthening alternatives and skills (such as a better capacity to mentalize both self and others).
- To build a mentalizing community and with it a secure base for exploration of thoughts and feelings regarding one's own and others' mental states in the context of relationships.
- To facilitate the expression of difficult affects and explore the individual meaning of the experience of chronic illness.

The MBTG-A approach emphasizes the sharing of thoughts and feelings in the context of everyday social situations. Exchanges in the group allow for consideration of cultural understanding and relevant individual values (e.g. ethnic traditions, spiritual beliefs) and are respectful and attentive to the personal meaning of the experience. Furthermore, this approach does not follow a pre-packaged set of exercises. Rather, it is meant to be a playground of ideas and an exchange of experiences guided by basic aims in the facilitators' minds. However, certain activities have proven especially useful in promoting the aims of the groups such as the use of popular television programmes which illustrate stressful interpersonal circumstances, as these allow the group (especially during early stages) to explore difficult issues of displacement.

For example, during our renal group the discussion of the show *Big Brother* provided a wonderful opportunity to explore participants' beliefs around interpersonal relationships. There was particular interest in the issue of being excluded, the group's participants identification with the people ousted from the *Big Brother* house and their feelings of being misunderstood and unfairly treated. The members of the renal group were also able to make a link between the lack of privacy in our group and the *Big Brother* experience, bringing to the fore difficult feelings regarding being 'public property of the medical staff'.

Technical issues such as the duration of the group, the nature of the group (closed vs. open) and the use of one or two facilitators are often determined by the needs of group participants and the logistics of the setting. For example, when working in a small hospital unit, one has less control over the age difference between attending group members, whereas at a school site, it is easier to form separate groups based on gender and age differences if required. The average group lasts from eight to 12 sessions. Based on the experience of recent applications, the group should not be bigger than eight members. This size allows the group facilitator(s) to get to know members and to be able to keep in mind the unspoken group processes and the sequences of interacting, thinking and feeling that take place in the group. Furthermore, it allows enough time for a basic structure which includes the use of an ice-breaker, free-floating discussion and at times more structured skill-based activities.

As mentioned earlier, the group leaders serve as facilitators and models of mentalizing. So, like the mother who tries to figure out why the baby cries, the facilitators acknowledge out loud their own concerns about people not knowing what to do or say; or venture into modelling behaviours such as guessing what people might be feeling or thinking, or begin by sharing some of their own concerns, and put themselves in a non-expert position which allows them to wonder and invite others to do so. As a result, there is a horizontal approach in which the facilitators share their own experiences and reflect on their own non-mentalizing impasses during the group. This stance is particularly helpful in the context of the hospital unit where the needs of the body (concrete) often overshadow the emotional and social ones (abstract).

The group discussed in this chapter was facilitated by only one professional (the author) due to logistical constraints. However, I strongly feel, based on further experience, that a co-facilitator approach is more effective in promoting mentalization by providing the opportunity for modelling of mentalizing in action by the facilitating pair. For example, when the group encounters a 'mentalizing impasse', the facilitating pair is able to reflect with each other and illustrate the skills which promote effective mentalization.

Regarding dynamics within the group, the focus remains on pointing out the use of maladaptive defensive strategies when encountered within the group, followed by the introduction of mentalizing techniques such as 'checking' and 'stop-and-rewind' (Fonagy & Bateman, 2006) in order to facilitate a 'mentalizing exchange'. In summary, the aim is to create a community where the focus is on mentalizing and identifying what inhibits its functioning for each individual and the group. In other words, the group aims to offer a 'new developmental experience' conducive to new ways of thinking about feelings in the context of relationships.

Difficulties in mentalizing interpersonal stress in an adolescent renal unit

A brief illustration

Before starting a mentalization-based group in the paediatric haemodialysis unit, the author spent a period observing in the hospital setting, in order to better understand the processes surrounding the experience of living with chronic kidney failure from diagnosis to transplantation. Observation of outpatient follow-up meetings between doctors, young people and their caregivers took place as well as observation in all units of the paediatric nephrology department. The following extract describes an interaction observed during this initial period:

It is 7 am on a Saturday morning and the nurses of the haemodialysis unit are getting ready for another hectic morning. They move around as the roaring sounds and smells of the machines in the unit awaken the senses of the incoming patients, doctors and visitors. Suddenly, Jane, one of the adolescents receiving treatment, walks in. She looks unwell, dishevelled, dragging her feet as she enters the unit. Mary, a nurse in the unit, greets her and makes a joke about her appearance, asking if the party last night was good. I understand this as an effort on Mary's part to make positive contact and try to relate to Jane in a casual manner, as if indicating 'I come in peace', since their relationship has often been quite tense and difficult. Jane mumbles a comment: 'Some nurse you are, I am sick, I have a fever you. . .'. Mary makes eye contact with me as the exchange is going on next to my chair near the weight scale. Mary speaks to me: 'See what I have to deal with here?' I smile empathically and remain quiet. Jane asks if she can be in the sick room, she is in no mood for chatting today. Mary replies that this can be arranged.

Suddenly, the room is taken over by the sounds of Mary and Jane arguing in the sick room. Jane refuses to stand on the scale and extend her arm for a blood pressure check. Mary speaks loudly about Jane's lack of self care and the consequences of her irresponsible behaviour on her health. Jane puts her earphones on. The scene is filled with tense silences and facial threats thereafter. Mary comes out of the room and goes into the nurses' break room to speak to an incoming young doctor who has been paged due to Jane's fever. Jane becomes more contained with the doctor, with whom she seems to communicate better, and Mary becomes manically busy and eventually goes into the nurses' lounge to have a cup of tea and speaks to a colleague about her feelings of anger and frustration.

(Research Observation Log)

The above took place during the early days of my observation and illustrates a unique stressor interfering with the capacity of this system to mentalize, i.e. the constant reminder of the fragility of a failing young body. Mary, feeling helpless and frustrated with Jane's ongoing lack of cooperation, chooses to try to scare Jane by reminding her of all the bad things that are going to happen to her if she continues to consume so many liquids daily. I witnessed an almost complete failure of the capacity to mentalize as both parties were overwhelmed by their feelings.

What we seek to promote with the mentalization-based group is to elicit such interactions in the group and to invite the participants to think about possible reasons why one might behave in this way, which are not immediately obvious. For this purpose, we introduce the concept of 'opaqueness of states of mind'. For example, if we were to discuss Jane's reaction, we would invite Mary to be part of our discussion and introduce a 'guessing' activity in which we promote within the group an atmosphere where a potentially stressful situation can be prevented by 'checking' with the other about what they guess might be the thoughts and feelings causing the relational impasse.

As illustrated by the vignette, the lack of privacy and the young people's sense of being 'public property' is something that needs to be addressed with staff, family members and participants. It is very important to reach an agreement as to when the group feels they need to have a certain level of privacy while discussing issues. This is often not so easy to achieve in a medical setting as things are often unpredictable and several emergencies may occur, so it is important to reflect on this situation and take advantage of the opportunity to explore participants' feelings. For example, it is very likely that Jane's reaction had to do with past experiences of being reprimanded in front of others for her incapacity to control liquids adequately.

So, in this context, a mentalization-based intervention seeks to promote systemic change as much as to elicit progressive individual developmental strides in the group. Including the nursing and medical staff and providing them with the opportunity to mentalize about their own feelings regarding adherence and overall response to adolescent behaviour is key in the process of affecting environmental change that will recognize and encourage the young person's mentalizing efforts.

In this context, non-adherence to medical regime can be understood as a non-mentalizing response to the fear of being engulfed by the illness and as a developmentally appropriate need to feel independent and in control of one's body and one's actions. However, these feelings of agency are quickly substituted by fear and anger over the reality of having a young person's body with baby needs, resulting in higher levels of depression in this population as indicated in the literature (Brownbridge & Fielding, 1994).

A mentalization-based group in the adolescent renal unit

The renal group met for 12 sessions on Saturday mornings. This was a small but diverse group with two boys and four girls from African, Asian and European backgrounds. Out of the six young people attending our group, four manifested chronic histories of non-adherence to medical regime. As a result, two of them had failed transplants and were not placed back on the transplantation waiting list.

As part of the initial assessment, all six young people were invited to complete the Millon Adolescent Personality Interview (MAPI) (Millon *et al.*, 1984). All participants were found to meet criteria for at least one diagnostic category according to *DSM IV-R* (as assessed by the MAPI). The most frequent diagnosis was adjustment disorder with mixed emotional features or with depressed mood. Half of the group's participants indicated they experienced significant levels of dissatisfaction with self-esteem and social tolerance. Preoccupations with peer security and self-concept were apparent in three out of six young people while only one participant showed significant problems with body image. Overall, there was a strong preoccupation with social and peer issues, underlying once more the importance of the relational dimension for this population.

Before the group began several meetings had taken place with medical staff regarding the aims of the intervention as well as in order to discuss the concept of mentalization. On the basis of these discussions, unit nurses were asked to remain away from the group area during 'discussion time', which lasted from one hour to an hour and a half depending on medical emergencies or doctors' visits. Young people were also encouraged to ask their companions (siblings, parents and friends) to step out during sessions and issues of confidentiality were often discussed and decided upon from session to session, so an open and flexible approach was adopted. The group always began with the same ice-breaker, in which participants reported something good and something bad which had happened to them that week. After that, a new theme based on an initial survey of group participants was introduced and discussed. Often, a ten-minute psychoeducational module was included in which the facilitator invited group members to be part of an activity that highlighted a new concept such as a mentalizing technique or the concept of mentalization itself. Group members were constantly encouraged to explore their feelings in the here-and-now and inquire about the feelings of others in the group.

When thinking of coping strategies, the group was often invited to create their own language and shared words they could use to understand their behaviour. For instance, when thinking about the topic of adherence one of the young women explained that non-adherence was 'a stupid but effective way of getting noticed', so we explored together not only other ways of being heard and listened to but also the emotional states that often motivated non-adherent behaviour. This topic often emerged when a stressful situation had occurred prior to the group during the pre-monitoring period of the haemodialysis session, like the one described earlier between Jane and Mary.

So, was the mentalization-based group helpful to a young woman like Jane who had endured the experience of a failing body since a young age? In fact, Jane's acceptance of the group was vital for the other young people in the unit as she held a privileged position both as the oldest and also as the member of the unit who acted out her feelings of frustration and anger most openly. In fact, her active, almost hypervigilant inquisitiveness facilitated the introduction of the concept of mentalization and its playful discussion at the beginning of the group. During this initial discussion, it became clear to me that Jane was actually too good a mentalizer and because of this, she struggled to join others in what she perceived as a clumsy and disrespectful attempt to understand her behaviour. She had grown up as a parentified child and as a result she was extremely skilful at reading grown-up cues and challenging their vulnerabilities when she felt, in her own words, 'cornered' or misunderstood. This tendency emerged frequently in the group, particularly during a discussion about our relationship with our bodies:

One of the boys in the group challenged Jane's hope of obtaining a transplant and having kids and a normal life. Thirteen-year-old Tahir expressed his honest bewilderment at the thought of Jane wanting to put her body through the effort and the pain of childbearing and birth after everything one has to endure when having sick kidneys. Feeling misunderstood and quite offended by Tahir's comment, Jane fired back by questioning his masculinity and his capacity to 'produce babies'. At this point, I stopped the interaction and proceeded to highlight the fact that something had happened and put forward my own questions regarding what had just happened and linked it to previous similar situations. Then I invited other group members to share their thoughts and feelings. The process of coming to a collective understanding of the conflict between two members included the exploration of both Tahir's and Jane's perspectives as well as a direct invitation to share their own understanding and experiences around this issue.

(Facilitator's Log)

By keeping our intervention in the here-and-now and by creating a mentalizing secure base within the group, we provided an opportunity for both Tahir and Jane to experience explicit mentalizing. Jane was able to speak about her fear of being misunderstood and being stuck in 'the sick girl role' for the rest of her life. She further explored her belief that by challenging her wish of becoming a mother Tahir was implying her body was rubbish, not able to produce a healthy baby. For Tahir, this was an opportunity to think about his own relationship with his body (with the support of the other young people in the unit), which he often ignored and denied. Together, the group was able to help Jane and Tahir think about strong feelings whilst still experiencing them. As a result, a sense of agency seemed to emerge around a painful issue and perhaps also an increasing awareness of the non-mentalizing strategies which often left them feeling frustrated and helpless, as was the case in the interactions between Jane and the nursing staff.

Some other themes that emerged during our intervention included: dealing with anger when faced with the demands of parents and peers; feelings around looking much younger; dealing with conflicts with friends and specifically boyfriends and girlfriends; learning to negotiate and speak out when feeling bullied; and concerns about transplants and the future. The theme of loss was quite prevalent as two group members were near the time of being transferred to an adult unit. Another topic that brought a great deal of non-mentalizing exchanges was the issue of different cultures: family, ethnic and medical culture and how they clash in the context of chronic illness. Discussing these issues from a mentalizing stance facilitated in the group the development of more coherent narratives around a highly disorganizing experience.

Evaluation of the intervention

Biological measures

Prior to the intervention a baseline of three indicators of medical adherence (weight, calcium and potassium) was established in order to follow the progression of adherence behaviour during the intervention and six months after it was completed. Findings of these measures indicated a general reduction in the number of excessive weight gain observations between the baseline period (prior to the intervention) and subsequent periods in all participants. This improvement was still observed six months after the end of the intervention.

Findings regarding adherence to calcium medication indicated no clear pattern across participants. Three participants showed significant improvement in adherence to calcium intake during the follow-up period in contrast to their inter-session measures during the intervention. Potassium indicators did not change significantly in any of the participants.

In sum, the findings from the biological markers of outcome were somewhat mixed. One must remember that biological measures of renal patients are influenced by a diverse number of variables specific to each patient's condition. Nevertheless, all participants showed an increased understanding of the motivation behind their non-adherent behaviour during discussions, and this was particularly true of the issue of liquid intake, which seems to be largely confirmed by our measures.

Pilot mentalization assessment

A computerized instrument showing six vignettes, three telling stories that depict stressful interpersonal conflicts that the average adolescent encounters (non-context) and three specific to the experiences of being chronically ill (context), were administered before and after the intervention in order to assess the style and functioning of mentalization as well as frequently used coping strategies. In addition, the performance of each renal group participant was compared to that of a healthy child (control) of his or her gender and age. In three out of six cases we found that the performance of the control pairs was higher than that of the renal participants on the pre-test responses. However, we found that the performance of the renal participants was closer to that of the paired controls in context-related questions than in non-context related questions. That is, young people suffering from ESRD were more mentalizing when presented with vignettes related to the experience of being chronically ill, underlying perhaps the organizing quality of the experience of illness in the development of self in the context of relationships.

Second, the performance of each renal participant was compared between the pre- and the post-tests, again separately averaging the scores across the six non-context and the six context questions. Most renal participants (five out of six) showed improved performance on this measure between the pre- and post-tests. The average improvement in performance was higher for the non-context than for the context questions. That is, young people with renal disease improved on average more in their capacity to mentalize when presented with vignettes illustrating interpersonal conflicts which were not directly related to the experience of being chronically ill.

In this study no attachment measure was included in the assessment battery, but it would be important for further research to include existing attachment tools as this could inform further ways in which attachment influences the capacity to cope effectively with the experience of chronic illness.

In general, it appears that a relationally focused group approach seems to be more meaningful than an individual intervention in the context of a medical unit as it has a greater potential to influence supportive systems around the young person. However, there are significant challenges when it comes to maintaining confidentiality and providing a strong base for further replication of the intervention carried out by professionals working in the unit, as this is an unpredictable and ever-changing environment where relationships are fragile and often stress is heightened by the very difficult nature of the job: keeping a young person alive.

Conclusion

Clinical work with chronically ill adolescents and their families is an area where the psychodynamically oriented professional can offer insight and help develop meaningful interventions. The mentalization-based group approach provides a very promising framework for this work with its flexible and playful structure whilst still being grounded in a strong theoretical base. However, in order to accomplish the process of integration and translation into effective community-based interventions we must become aware first of how our personal and professional knowledge and experiences inform our own relational styles and capacities. In this way, the mentalizing therapist wears her ability to think and feel not as armour but as a walking and hearing aid in the process of trying to understand the young people she hopes to help.

Embarking on such a reflective journey by listening to the diversity of discourses among the young people in the group will help the therapist to decide which themes will be relevant and effective in fostering the mentalizing capacities of a specific population. This is especially true when working with young people who have experienced trauma in order to allow for the expression and even reinforcement of desirable human relational capacities such as trust, intimacy, care and community. In this manner, the mentalizing therapist seeks to offer new ways of articulating basic aspects of self experience, thus a higher quality of emotional life.

Furthermore, by maintaining a position of 'not knowing' the mentalizing therapist remains curious about the stories that the group members tell. This curiosity helps her to ask questions and respond in ways that enable patients and families to expand the domain of the not-yet-said in their own chronic illness situation. When we invite the young people we work with to tell and retell, write and rewrite the narratives of their illness and life journeys under the auspices of the mentalizing and containing group environment, new meanings may emerge that often help young people and their families move past stuck points or enter periods of transition and change.

References

Anderson, B., Ho, J., Brackett, J., Finkelstein, D., & Laffel, L. (1997). Parental involvement in diabetes management tasks: Relationships to blood glucose monitoring adherence and metabolic control in young adolescents with insulin-dependent diabetes mellitus. *Journal of Paediatrics*, 130, 257–265.

Bergmann, T., & Freud, A. (1965). *Children in the hospital* (p. 151). New York: International Universities Press.

Brownbridge, G., & Fielding, D. M. (1994). Psychosocial adjustment and adherence to dialysis treatment regimes. *Paediatric Nephrology*, 8, 744–749.

Burroughs, T. E., Pontious, S. I., & Santiago, J. V. (1993). The relationship among six psychosocial domains, age, health care adherence, and metabolic control in adolescents with IDDM. *Diabetic Education*, 19, 396–402.

Clay, D. L., Mardhorst, M. J., & Lehn, L. (2002). Empirically supported treatments in pediatric psychology: Where is the diversity? *Journal of Pediatric Psychology*, 27(4), 325–337.

Curtin, R. B., Svarstad, B. L., & Keller, T. H. (1999). Haemodialysis patient's non-compliance with oral medication. *American Nephrology Nurses Association*, 26, 307–316.

Fonagy, P., & Bateman, A. (2006). *Mentalization-based treatment for borderline personality disorder: A practical guide* (pp. 133–135). Oxford: Oxford University Press.

Fonagy, P., & Moran, G. (1990). Studies on the efficacy of child psychoanalysis. *Journal of Consulting and Clinical Psychology*, 58, 684–695.

Freud, A. (1952). The role of bodily illness in the mental life of children. In *The Writings of Anna Freud*, Vol. IV. New York: International Universities Press, 1968.

Garralda, M. E., Jameson, R. A., Reynolds, J. M., & Postlethwaite, R. J. (1988). Psychiatric adjustment in children with chronic renal failure. *Journal of Child Psychology & Psychiatry*, 29, 79–90.

Haberbeck-Weber, C., & McKee D. H. (1995). Prevention of emotional and behavioural distress in children experiencing hospitalization and chronic illness. In M. C Robert (Ed.), *Handbook of paediatric psychology* (pp. 167–184). New York: Guilford Press.

Henning, P., Tomlinson, L., Rigden, S. P., & Haycock, G. B. (1988). Long term outcome of treatment of end stage renal failure. *Archives of Disease in Childhood*, 63, 35–40.

Kazdin, A. E., & Weisz, J. R. (1998). Identifying and developing empirically supported child and adolescent treatments. *Journal of Consulting and Clinical Psychology*, 66, 19–36.

Kyngas, H., Kroll, T., & Duffy, M. E. (2000). Compliance in adolescents with chronic diseases: A review. *Journal of Adolescent Health*, 26, 379–388.

Leggat, J. E., Orzol, S. M., & Hulbert-Shearon, T. E. (1998). Non-compliance in haemodialysis: Predictors and survival analysis. *American Journal of Kidney Disorders*, 32, 139–145.

Malberg, N. T., Fonagy, P., & Mayes, L. (2008). Contemporary psychoanalysis in a pediatric hemodialysis unit: Development of a mentalization-based group intervention for adolescent patients with end-stage renal disease. *The Annual of Psychoanalysis*, 36, 101–114.

Millon, T., Green, C., & Meagher, R. (1984). *Millon Adolescent Personality Inventory*. Minneapolis, MN: Interpretive Scoring Systems.

National Kidney and Urologic Diseases Information Clearinghouse (NKUDIC, 2010). Kidney failure. Available HTTP: http://wwww.kidney.niddk.nih.gov (accessed October 15 2010).

Plante, W. A., Lobato, D., & Engel, R. (2001). Review of group interventions for pediatric chronic conditions. *Journal of Pediatric Psychology*, 26, 435–453.

Poursanidou, K., Graner, P., Watson, A., & Stephenson, R. (2003). Difficulties and support at school for children following renal transplantation: Health professionals' views. Paper presented at the British Educational Research Association Annual Conference, Edinburgh.

Ramsden, S. (1999). The child and adolescent psychotherapist in the community. In M. Lanyado & A. Horne (Eds.), *Child and adolescent psychotherapy: Psychoanalytic approaches* (pp. 141–158). London and New York: Routledge.

Reynolds, J. M., Garralda, M. E., Jameson, R. A., & Postlethwaite, R. J. (1986). Living with chronic renal failure. *Child Care Health Development*, 12, 401–407.

Soliday, E., Kool, E., & Lande, M. (2000). Psychosocial adjustment in children with kidney disease. *Journal of Pediatric Psychology*, 25, 93–103.

Swartz, A. L. (1998). Adherence in children with renal disease. In L. B. Myers & K. Midence (Eds.), *Adherence to treatment in medical conditions* (p. 455). Amsterdam: Harwood.

Chapter 9

Supporting and enhancing mentalization in community outreach teams working with hard-to-reach youth

The AMBIT approach

Dickon Bevington and Peter Fuggle

Introduction

This chapter describes a newly developed mentalizing approach known as adolescent mentalization-based integrative therapy (AMBIT) which has been designed for teams who work with young people who are often referred to as 'hard-to-reach', on account of the fact that conventional clinic-based services are poorly suited to serve their needs. The purpose of this chapter is to outline some of the key aspects of this approach, particularly with respect to its focus on supporting and nurturing mentalizing capacities within an AMBIT team.

The chapter has three sections: first, we describe the context of working with hard-to-reach young people and how this presents specific challenges to developing an evidence-based approach; second, we provide a brief overview of the core components of the AMBIT model – what we call the 'AMBIT stance'; third, we outline three core practices used by team members to support mentalization within their work and in the team process.

Context – the nature of work with hard-to-reach young people

Hard-to-reach young people

From a welfare perspective these young people may be described as hard-to-reach, whereas for other sections of society they are anything but hard to reach: drug dealers, gangs, delinquent peers and other exploitative adults find them readily accessible. Finding ways of working that might provide some competitive edge over the immediacy of what these negative influences in their social ecology offer (for instance, safety, albeit that the safety a dealer offers is contingent and likely to be time limited) is a key challenge. A local dealer or gang leader may be in a markedly more powerful position than a local service seeking to influence the dire trajectories that these hard-to-reach youth often describe, as they move towards the more entrenched positions of adulthood.

Complexity

Hard-to-reach young people commonly have a life trajectory shaped by multiple and cumulative burdens and risks rather than a single issue such as mental illness. Whilst a high proportion will have mental health problems, including developmental disorders such as attention deficit hyperactivity disorder (ADHD), post-traumatic symptoms, anxiety and depression, self-injurious behaviours, and not uncommonly emerging mental states in relation to psychosis and poorly adaptive personality organization, most will also have co-morbidities in the form of substance use disorders, conduct disorder or delinquency, offending, and educational failure. To add to this, hard-to-reach youth tend to have families that are either unable (due to parental ill health, low parenting skills or poverty) or unwilling (due to negative past experience of the care system in the parents themselves or cultural biases against engaging with services) to assist or insist upon the young person accessing what professionals might consider to be appropriate care.

Epidemiological studies (e.g. Kessler *et al.*, 2010) demonstrate a significant cohort of youth for whom it is the very complexity that conspires to produce the poorest prognoses, and which most powerfully undermines the effectiveness of interventions occurring in single domains. For example, the young person may present in such a way that, individually, he or she may fail to pass diagnostic or operational thresholds of 'caseness', which means that services set up to deliver problem-specific help may themselves fail to offer help, framing the presenting problem as being outside their remit. Where appointments are offered but are not attended, a busy clinic may understandably assume that the family or child no longer has need of this help, or that their limited resources are best directed at problems more likely to respond to the interventions they are able to offer.

The Tower of Babel effect

Frequently such young people fall into the spaces between services, or are offered multiple assessments that result in little effective action. Alternatively, it is not uncommon for young people to have a nominal engagement with multiple services, perhaps with named workers from social care, mental health, youth offending and educational services, or more. The engagement in such cases may be nominal because of another problem that we refer to as the 'Tower of Babel' effect. The multiple workers from different training backgrounds will likely use different models of intervention based on different explanatory models (neurobiological, social ecological, cognitive-behavioural, systemic, psychodynamic, to name but five), and naturally workers tend to frame a young person's or their family's difficulties, implicitly or explicitly, in the language of their own training. Given that more than a century of research into the behavioural sciences has signally (and quite properly, given the complexity referred to above) failed to deliver an overarching 'super-theory' that embraces all forms of help, it is not surprising that families and young people who are at their most fragmented frequently fail to integrate the input they receive, and instead experience this, rightly or wrongly, as either contradictory or intentionally unhelpful.

Now many, probably most, hard-to-reach young people have disturbed attachment histories, and struggle to activate any kind of secure internal working model of attachment that would support them in taking the risky step of placing trust in a worker. Just as mentalizing capacity of the carer is linked to security of attachment in the child, so we find that the mentalizing capacities of these young people are often compromised and restricted, in the face of frequent activation or disorganization of their attachment systems (Fonagy & Target, 2005). In addition, being required to form multiple attachments to multiple workers, who may appear to be in disagreement, or even openly contradict one another, may only serve to exacerbate this.

Because of the risky and often antisocial behaviour of many of these young people, it is understandable that workers from different agencies may either experience high levels of threat from the young people or have severe anxieties about their welfare and safety. For engaged practitioners both of these mental states tend to compromise their own capacity to accurately mentalize the predicaments of their clients, being driven instead into increasingly assertive or even coercive relationships, or to abandon the young person via the process of onwards referral. The net result is that the wider system, out of the best of intentions, strives to deliver highly specialized interventions, but paradoxically, and too often, delivers a service that is experienced at best as ineffective and at worst as aversive. Finally, given the above, it is no surprise to find that the threat of therapeutic nihilism (in clients, and in the wider care network) is another hurdle for practitioners to overcome in addressing themselves to this group.

Building on the evidence

Current approaches to working with hard-to-reach young people

Fortunately, much ground has already been travelled in developing services for this group. AMBIT acknowledges this, and seeks to build on the existing evidence base. Two interventions, namely multisystemic therapy (MST; Henggeler & Borduin, 1990) and multidimensional family therapy

(MDFT; Liddle *et al.*, 2001) deserve particular mention as exemplary in their labours to test their efforts in valid trials.

Multisystemic therapy was originally developed as a treatment for conduct-disordered and delinquent youth, and takes a radically social-ecological and multisystems approach, emphasizing work with the multiple systems around the young person and his or her family, to some extent above direct face-to-face working. MST offers a clear, manualized framework to structure and prioritize goals within which a range of evidence-based interventions (mainly drawn from systemic or cognitive-behavioural models of treatment) are deployed. In a series of trials that are impressive, given the challenge that research with this population poses, this approach has indicated effectiveness mainly in reducing offending, but also across a range of wider social, educational and mental health outcomes (e.g. Henggeler *et al.*, 2003), although recent meta-analyses have questioned its superiority to other forms of intervention (Littell *et al.*, 2005). More recently, MST has extended its reach into more explicit mental health arenas, and to work with child abuse and neglect. There is again some trials evidence of effectiveness in these arenas, although without (as yet) the robust highly clinically-significant replicated outcomes that support its original remit. In addition to its evidenced support for carefully manualized approaches, with attention to fidelity to a treatment model, MST also demonstrates that a single worker, supported by a robust supervisory framework and skilled in a range of different evidence-based interventions, can be an effective agent of change in this complex territory.

On the other hand MST and its variants, in its admirable focus on developing evidence, has necessarily had to introduce quite significant exclusion criteria which mean that the hardest to reach young people may not be included in trials; for instance, presentations with psychosis, homelessness, or non-family placements, or institutional placements (e.g. Swenson *et al.*, 2010). This is potentially problematic for a team delivering a pragmatic ('take what comes') service, rather than a selective one. MST does not place a high emphasis on the relationship between young person and worker, rather emphasizing the need for engagement at the level of the family and wider system. The large majority of MST trials have been conducted with young people/families who are in some sense, formally or informally, mandated into treatment, and this does not necessarily address the needs of the hard-to-reach, whose very capacity to keep one step ahead of services (including law enforcement) is a significant part of the problem. In the view of AMBIT, this necessitates a high focus on the skills of workers to make and sustain voluntary engagements with the young people and their networks – the mentalization-based approach to work offers a framework for this.

Multidimensional family therapy is pre-eminently a multimodal approach, which has also developed some evidence of effectiveness in randomized trials, most of which involve working with hard-to-reach populations, such as runaway and/or drug-using youth (Liddle *et al.*, 2001). Some of the detailed process research that has accompanied randomized trials and effectiveness research in MDFT has highlighted the value of maintaining a balance of active intervention across multiple domains of functioning as being critical to good outcomes (Hogue *et al.*, 2006). It seems that uni-modal therapies that address single domains (for example, the inner world of motivation, cognitions, or of the family system) appear less effective than approaches that systematically address themselves to multiple domains.

Challenges to implementation of effective practice

So, although there is hard-won progress, and clear pointers towards factors associated with effective practice exist, there remain many unanswered questions, and for this client group the evidence base remains weak in relation to the question of 'what works for whom?'.

Costs aside, if training is available, there are further hurdles for a service trying to implement an evidence-based, manualized treatment. First, there is evidence that practitioners not uncommonly dislike working to manualized protocols (Addis & Krasnow, 2000). Workers report a sense of frustration at the implications that come with the top-downwards delivery of instructions from 'silos of expertise' that may be far removed from the site of action. At the risk of over-generalization, workers drawn to the kind of work may have a common presenting feature, which is a belief in the value of flexibility and individual creativity in developing relationships and demonstrating contingency in their response to the demands of the young people they are working with. Such workers struggle with what they may perceive as too rigid a format. Whilst the evidence from outcomes research is clearly not on the side of 'free-form benign eclecticism', a position that protects some of this adaptive flexibility may have value. We believe that there is value in an approach that attempts to plot a middle path between two methods of work that are caricatured (unfairly) as 'therapy-by-numbers' or unstructured 'do-it-yourself' approaches.

Second, expertise that is delivered from afar may be poorly attuned to the precise cultural, demographic, geographical or wider systemic demands of the local setting, let alone the question of whether it addresses local variations in psychopathology. In the field of substance use disorders, for instance, new drugs increasingly arise in the field, and are propagated so fast that specific manualized approaches to the treatment needs relating to these specific substances may struggle to keep up. More generally, as the evidence base for effectiveness moves forwards, paper manuals may become rapidly outdated, and can serve as 'anchors', resisting change towards best practice, rather than enhancing it.

As large books, or files, treatment manuals are not portable, and are less frequently consulted than they could or should be, particularly if they are to influence practice on the ground. Too often they serve more to define the 'what' in the mind of the commissioners paying for a service, rather than the actual service that the therapeutic team is delivering. It is difficult to measure the role that appreciation and utilization of local expertise has to play in sustaining a sense of self-efficacy in a team, but in the authors' view this is likely to be important in building sustainable teams.

The basic stance of AMBIT

The AMBIT approach seeks to address some of the challenges described above. First, AMBIT is fundamentally a team approach, which aims to be of relevance to a range of teams working with hard-to-reach young people, whether in the public or voluntary sector. It is not a therapy that an individual practitioner could implement on their own or within a wider non-AMBIT team.

The intention is that all workers within an AMBIT team should adopt a similar basic stance in their work, and this is outlined in this section. This basic stance consists of eight descriptors of an ideal 'intentional therapeutic stance' for keyworkers (see Figure 9.1). We conceive of the eight indicators of the stance as operating like the 'grab rails' in a railway carriage: easy to reach out for in order to steady oneself and 'keep your head when all about you are losing theirs' (Kipling, 1910).

This stance recognizes that non-standard (outreach) settings for therapy, and the dilemmas that this client group tends to bring, often generate high anxiety in the worker, so that one of the starting points for AMBIT is how one may generate, sustain and share best practice in such an environment. We know that high affect, or more specifically arousal of the threat-avoidance or attachment systems, inhibits explicit mentalizing (Fonagy *et al.*, 2004), which reduces the worker's effectiveness. This is why at the heart of AMBIT is a dialectical notion: on the one hand attention is paid to developing or supporting an individual therapeutic attachment relationship between a keyworker and the young person (one that activates 'secure internal working models' and helps to repair, stimulate, or sustain mentalizing in the young person); on the other hand there is a strong focus on team working – shifting away from the conventional 'team around the child' configuration, towards a 'team around the worker' (see Figure 9.2). Crucially, other team members must see the disciplined support they provide for their colleagues' own mentalizing, as being core to their working practices, rather than as something that is superfluous to their main task.

The eight descriptors of an ideal 'intentional therapeutic stance' for keyworkers are as follows:

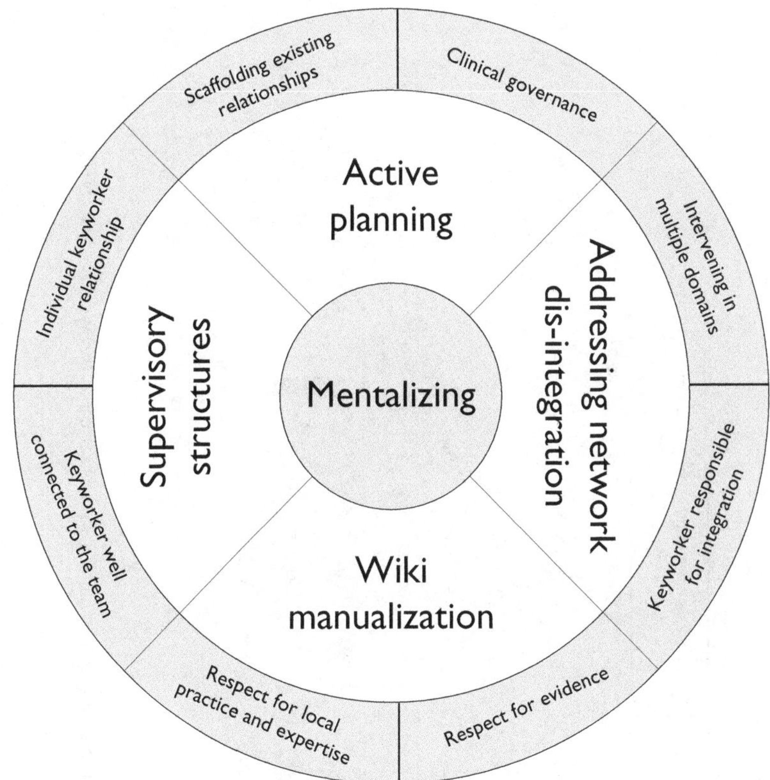

Figure 9.1 AMBIT stance and basic practice

a) Individual keyworker relationship
b) Well-connected team
c) Intervening in multiple domains
d) Taking responsibility for integration
e) Scaffolding existing relationships
f) Clinical governance
g) Respect for local expertise
h) Respect for evidence

Individual keyworker relationship

Key to stimulating, repairing, and sustaining mentalizing function in a young person is the development of something approaching secure attachment with a trusted figure, who can be experienced by the young person as having their mind 'in mind'.

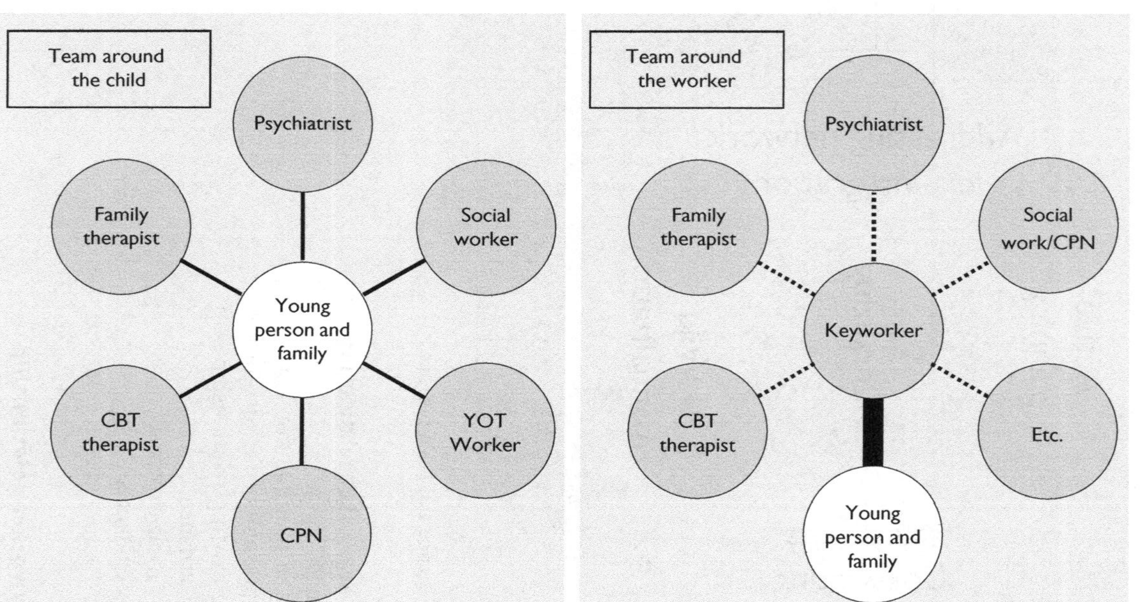

Figure 9.2 AMBIT: a shift of emphasis – actively stimulating and sustaining mentalization in the worker colleague as a core team task

Well-connected team

Nowhere is the organizational emphasis in the implementation of mentalizing practice clearer than in the notion of the 'well-connected team'. This refers to the concept that, at its most basic, practitioners retain close and frequent communication with each other, actively attending to each others' mentalizing, despite frequently operating as single outreach workers. They use basic technology such as mobile phones to facilitate this, but also use clear, and to an extent 'ritualized', social disciplines to structure the way they conduct discussion, one of which ('Thinking Together') is described below (pp. 176–180).

Intervening in multiple domains

By domains we refer to the different territories upon and within which symptoms and interventions are played out; from the molecular and physiological, through individual psychological, family and systemic, and out to the wider social ecology including peer group and the complex multi-agency care and educational networks. As described above, it is the very complexity that conspires to produce the poorest prognosis, and which most powerfully undermines the effectiveness of interventions occurring in single domains. Treating a young person's depressive cognitions and low motivation to resist self-medication with cannabis is unlikely to be successful without addressing the fact that his mother is supplying the cannabis he smokes on the grounds that he is more biddable under its influence. Workers in an AMBIT service are expected to develop specific interventions in at least two separate functional domains. The kinds of individual interventions deployed are, wherever possible, manualized and evidence based; motivational, cognitive-behavioural, family interventions and work with the wider service ecology. As a general rule these individual modalities are integrated through the lens of mentalization.

Taking responsibility for integration

Taking seriously the young person's experience of and capacity to engage usefully with care is crucial to AMBIT. By 'care' we mean the totality of concerned and responsible adults attending to the global health, developmental and educational needs of the young person. We have described above how it is common for multiple workers and/or teams or agencies to be involved in delivering the different components of this care. Whereas in ordinary life this arrangement works well, and the separation of silos of experience carries many advantages, in complex and highly pathological cases there are corresponding drawbacks to this multiplication of workers, which we have characterized above as the 'Tower of Babel effect', and which can easily confound the best intentions of the network around any young person.

An AMBIT keyworker proactively predicts such difficulties and deploys a range of activities to limit the extent to which they may act as barriers to effective interventions. These might range from acting as a single multi-skilled 'jack of all trades (or 'barefoot') worker' in the earliest phase of engagement (when multiple relationships may be perceived as overwhelming) to working as an 'interpreter' to explain, contextualize and support the work of other professionals in the network, to more proactive attempts to identify and address dis-integration in the network (described below under the 'dis-integration grid').

Scaffolding existing relationships

Workers must direct their attention to identifying resiliencies in the young person's social ecology, recognizing the importance of strengthening existing relationships that are likely to persist considerably longer than any professional contact. We assume that referral for help, particularly requests for dramatic away-from-home solutions (hospitalization or social care), occur at the point at which the local ecosystem experiences itself as being overwhelmed. In this explicit effort to intervene at a systemic level within the young person's social ecology we draw upon the work of other evidence-based approaches such as MST and MDFT (see pp. 165–167). This acknowledges the paradoxical risk of degrading the sense of self-efficacy within the family and wider social ecology when well-intentioned professionals are seen as intervening from a position of expertise, contrasted to the assumed 'incompetence' of the family. At times this approach may require teams to accept the real over the ideal in terms of the quality of the relationships that we are called upon to scaffold. Notwithstanding adherence to proper safeguarding and child protection procedures we are mindful of the poor outcomes for children whose care is institutionalized, let alone the financial cost of this alternative.

Clinical governance

In work with a high-risk group it is anticipated that appropriate governance structures are an expected part of practice. AMBIT claims no innovation in this respect, but in keeping with many aspects of mentalizing practice does place an emphasis on moving practices from the implicitly assumed or tacitly agreed towards more explicit shared expectations. AMBIT does not seek to supplant or replace locally agreed governance protocols, but rather to ensure that these are supported from above and adhered to by workers.

Respect for local expertise

Work in a complex multi-agency setting carries certain predictable risks, one of which is the liability of workers from these various agencies to be constantly exposed to biased negative feedback about each other. One of the commoner ways by which people seek to engage new workers or teams is in outlining – perhaps exaggerating – the shortcomings of previous workers or other teams. Aside from the mild challenge implicit in such an introduction (demanding that I do not prove so disappointing as they have), there is also a seductive quality to these conversations; the critic of my 'rivals' promises me the opportunity to better my colleagues in, say, education or social care. However, this cuts both ways and my colleagues are just as likely to be in receipt of criticisms of my service themselves. The net effect is often persistent myths about different services which have a pernicious effect upon the inter-agency environment, fostering unmentalized 'certainty' about the shortcomings of our colleagues, and a corresponding failure to mentalize their own best efforts, or to act as an effective interpreter of their work to our clients. An explicit and collective refusal to be drawn into these subtly subversive conversations characterizes the AMBIT team.

'Respect for local expertise' is also manifested in AMBIT insofar as it does not take a rigid 'one size fits all' approach to the precise form in which implementation takes place. Rigid insistence on deploying precise forms of practice that may have been developed in settings that are geographically and culturally distinct from the new service setting is something that can alienate the existing service ecology. Experienced local practitioners may resist adapting locally evolved expertise to fit a new service that may appear alien. Regardless of the rights or wrongs of this reaction, its effect appears to the authors to be a significant barrier to successful implementation.

Instead, AMBIT sets a basic stance, and expects local teams to become active to a greater or lesser extent in manualizing their own practice (see wiki manualization, pp. 183–184). Thus local teams over time form a composite of local expertise, that is integrated with a range of centrally derived and manualized specific interventions; these latter are generally evidence-based approaches which are integrated through the lens of mentalization. AMBIT trainings therefore start with a period of consultation through which the needs and demands upon the team are explicitly mentalized.

Respect for evidence

Just as mentalization sets the scene for what is to some extent merely a humble acceptance of the limits of one's knowing, so in relation to practice AMBIT emphasizes the need for a respectful stance towards the objective 'other's eye view' of validated scientific trials and evidence. Given our approach to the manualization of practice (see pp. 183–184) it is important to emphasize that AMBIT is not a free-for-all in which local teams are encouraged to 'make it up as they go along'. Instead, there is a realistic stance towards recognizing: (a) the relative paucity of robust trials evidence for work in this field; (b) the need to be scrupulous in gathering outcomes evidence in the work we do; and (c) the importance of using evidence-based practice where this does exist, although often this evidence has been gathered in far more controlled settings than an AMBIT team would generally be able to deploy it in.

From stance to practice in AMBIT

Collectively, the eight stance positions described above uphold five key aspects of practice:

1 Mentalizing.
2 Supervisory structures.
3 Addressing network dis-integration.
4 Active planning.
5 Wiki manualization.

Mentalizing

Mentalization is placed at the centre of AMBIT, recognizing its intrinsic value with respect to work with the young person and family/carers, but also as an integrative mechanism or lubricant that helps different component parts of the treatment, the team, and the wider network around the young person to work more coherently together. Thus, not only are the direct interventions with young people, their families and the wider social ecology directed towards stimulating and sustaining mentalization, but also mentalizing serves as a 'common currency' or language throughout the team. Specifically, workers in an AMBIT service should see their responsibility as being not only to increase or sustain mentalizing in their clients, but also in their professional colleagues.

To some extent, the next four key practice elements are designed to help resolve tensions that are inherent in upholding paired aspects of the stance that may often be experienced as contradictory.

Supervisory structures

Structures to facilitate oversight of each other's work are a fundamental aspect of AMBIT team practice, and emphasize the central importance of peer supervision as a process of supporting mentalization within the team; particularly called for (and supported by) the stance positions of *individual keyworker relationship* and *well-connected team*.

Addressing network dis-integration

This refers to the active commitment to work towards identifying and addressing significant dis-integration in the wider social and service network, as well as the more intimate dis-integration that a young person or their family may be experiencing. It is particularly called for (and supported by) the two stance positions intervening in multiple domains and taking responsibility for dis-integration. The use of simple tools such as the dis-integration grid (see Figure 9.3, p. 182) is an example of how this process can become proactive rather than reactive.

Active planning

This refers to the need for the AMBIT practitioner to be encouraged to have an explicit (intentional) purpose in all levels of the work with the young person, and with colleagues. This ranges from having a plan for a specific case discussion ('Thinking Together', see pp. 176–180) or contact with the young person, through having a plan for a specific session, to co-constructing (with the young person and carers) and maintaining overarching aims for the intervention as a whole. This practice will include considerations around managing risk, and developing a longer term trajectory of care, and is called for and supported by the stance positions of *scaffolding existing relationships* (some of which may carry risk) and *clinical governance*.

Wiki manualization

This is explained below (pp. 183–184), and refers to the fact that the treatment manual for AMBIT is explicitly designed as a collaborative integration of 'top-down' evidence-based material, with 'ground-up' local expertise.

Core AMBIT practices for maintaining mentalizing within a team

This section will describe three core AMBIT practices that are designed to sustain mentalizing functions within the team:

1 Thinking Together.
2 Mentalizing the network.
3 Manualizing the practice.

These core practices are highly practical and designed to be possible for teams working in pragmatic (and often under-resourced) community outreach settings. The intention is that these practices, with moderate levels of training, are also within the competencies of all staff working in such settings (independent of their professional background). In developing these practices, it is not required for a practitioner to have a therapy training background.

The assumption is that the nature of work with hard-to-reach young people presents a major challenge to retaining a mentalizing stance in the face of often severe adversity and a client group that have (at best) a very ambivalent relationship to help.

Thinking Together

As described earlier, AMBIT is a team-based approach to working with very troubled young people. This team approach is partly advocated in response to a number of common features about this work which make the maintenance of a mentalizing stance often hard to sustain. First, individual practitioners often work in physical isolation in community settings, doing home visits and meeting young people in a variety of community settings. Second, the young people may at times create considerable anxiety for the caseworker, either because of the risks that the young person is taking towards himself or herself and/or risks to others. Third, many young people are hard-to-reach in that they have a highly ambivalent or explicitly hostile relationship to help. This pattern of behaviour by the young person is likely to increase anxiety for the AMBIT caseworker.

All of these features lead to a potential loss of mentalizing for the caseworker in his or her work with the young person. For example, an AMBIT worker visits a young person at home and finds a situation in which the young person has just had a big row with her mother and has stormed out of the house saying she is going to kill herself. The parent is upset and angry. In such situations it may be difficult for the AMBIT worker to think clearly, to be able to find a reasonably relaxed, flexible stance and be able to mentalize readily about the parent's state of mind or that of the young person. There can be a tendency to move into non-mentalizing states such as teleological thinking (preoccupation with what to do) or with psychic equivalence (the belief that how the worker thinks/feels is actually how it is).

One of the starting points of AMBIT is that the loss of mentalizing in such situations is predictable and normal. This is emphasized in initial AMBIT training and there is explicit recognition that loss of mentalizing and high anxiety is not a position of shame for AMBIT workers. The whole approach focuses on team working that enables the AMBIT worker to re-establish a capacity to mentalize. This will enable the worker to think in a therapeutic way about the states of mind of the young person and his or her family before considering what actions may be needed in due course.

AMBIT strongly supports team members to share experience and discuss cases with each other, but to do so in the context of 'Active Planning' (see

p. 175) in order to get the best out of such interactions. In this way, team members are expected to support colleagues to think together about dilemmas and problems presented by the young people, which reduces isolation. Well-functioning teams do this as a matter of course and the AMBIT model explicitly promotes a sense of interdependency between team members, so that this is part of everyday practice, rather than an 'extra' to the daily work. This is very important in enabling team members to support each other in retaining a mentalizing stance. One of the key ways that mentalization can be reactivated is through contact and dialogue with an attachment figure (another member of the team), particularly one who is not in the centre of the anxieties around a particular case. Such conversations may take place in a number of different ways, such as by a phone call during a home visit to a colleague asking for advice, or informally between colleagues in the team office, as well as in supervision or team meetings.

However, in our view, although much case discussion takes place in most settings, not all conversations between colleagues result in improved mentalization of the particular dilemmas around a specific case. Due to the often highly volatile nature of the young people's life styles, these conversations can easily become narratives of recent 'dramatic' or high-risk events. This information sharing is often not productive and may paradoxically lead to amplified anxiety in the team, and particularly in the AMBIT caseworker. Dramatic and apparently exciting narratives of such events easily consume a lot of time and in our model are described as 'storytelling' (see below, p. 178). Storytelling does not necessarily lead to enhanced mentalizing for the caseworker.

AMBIT has developed a highly structured method of case discussion which aims primarily to enhance mentalization as a precursor to decision making and action. This practice is described as 'Thinking Together' and has four explicit steps. The clear intention of this method is that it can be followed equally easily in a wide range of contexts by phone or in person. We also recognize that such conversations often need to be brief. Our expectation is thinking together may often be carried out by team members in the ten minutes that they have spare for this issue.

Stage 1. Marking the task

The first stage is about explicit clarification of what is wanted out of the conversation, and is a short-term application of the practice of 'Active Planning'. '*What do you need from this conversation?*' is a good starting point. The task is for both the AMBIT worker and his or her colleague to work this out together and to be clear what is needed. In our experience, it is often this stage that is skipped past without having been worked out properly.

There are common conventions amongst mental health workers that it is useful to 'just talk it over' or 'just think with you about this'. This is understandable but such vague aims may indicate some degree of avoidance of actual thinking even when presented in the guise of thinking. In our view, thinking together does not happen easily and needs to start right from the beginning of the interchange. Using a formulaic naming of this exercise ('Thinking Together') serves to mark out the fact that this is to be a different kind of conversation – one which the colleague needs to 'contract' rather than 'drift' into. If this aspect of the conversation is not properly addressed, our prediction is that conversations easily drift back into story-telling. Having contracted in to 'Thinking Together', it is the responsibility of the colleague in this conversation to ensure that the AMBIT worker holds to the boundaries. This is sometimes quite hard. In some ways this can be seen as asking the keyworker to some degree to switch off biographical narrative memory and switch on reflective function. Examples of 'marking the task' at the start of a conversation are as follows:

> 'Okay, I'd like to think with you about how risky this young person is and whether the safety plan etc. is appropriate to the risks that he presents.'
>
> 'I don't know if I am making any progress with this case. I'd like to think with you to check whether the intervention plan needs to be changed.'
>
> 'I would like to think about what is going on in this young person's head. I can't work out why he is so hostile sometimes and so friendly some other times.'
>
> 'I really don't like his parents. I find it so difficult to be empathic to them. I'd like to think with you about why this might be happening.'

Stage 2. Stating the case

In the second stage, the AMBIT caseworker is encouraged to tell the key things that are relevant to the task that has been set. The catch phrase used in this stage is 'keeping to the bones' of the case relevant to the task. The aim and effort is directed at stimulating reflective descriptions rather than anecdotes of events and conversations that have occurred.

It is important for the AMBIT worker to mentalize what might be the 'simple bones' of the story or problem that their colleague might help with in the task that they have marked out together. There is never time to tell the whole story, so the colleague must act as a faithful editor, trying to represent to the best of his or her ability the account that has been given, but in an abbreviated form. Over-long storytelling is likely to be a version of non-mentalizing 'pretend mode' thinking. However, there is a balance to be struck between providing sufficient data and information to convey the richness and complexity of the story, and applying sufficient discernment to provide practical knowledge rather than an overwhelming 'sea of facts'.

The colleague has a duty to protect these boundaries and has effectively contracted to help the speaker keep to these boundaries. It may be necessary to point out: 'Hey, we need to keep to the simple bones here. . . is this getting into storytelling?' Equally the worker giving the account needs to hold onto this shared understanding of the task, so that such prompts are not taken as criticisms. Mentalization theory places error at the centre of communication – as something to be expected rather than it being a surprising disappointment. This is why some level of 'ritual' is emphasized in this exercise.

Stage 3. Mentalizing the moment

Having expressed the bones of the case, the AMBIT caseworker is invited explicitly to reflect on their own feelings about the case and the dilemma. The intention is to recognize present feelings of anger, anxiety or resentment that may be making it difficult to mentalize the caseworker's and the client's situation.

Another name for this is '*affective mentalization*', in some senses the highest order of mentalizing; that is, being able to feel a feeling and simultaneously to mentalize the experience. Feeling in the present tense may be a potential barrier to thinking, but, in awareness, it is also information for the practitioner. In this phase, worker and colleague are striving for that non-compulsive, tentative, hypothesizing and exploratory state of mind that characterizes active mentalizing – and which may often allow new formulations and potential actions to arise. Most importantly for this brief moment, the workers attempt to resist pressure compulsively to foreclose and shut down real thinking (perhaps on the grounds that the professionals know the answer, or that further thought is somehow indulgent and action is now required).

The theory of mentalization overlaps with cognitive-behavioural theory insofar as both assume that thinking and feeling interact together. This recognizes that my client's thoughts are influenced by his feelings and that my own attempts to weigh up the situation, the risks and the therapeutic direction are affected by my own affect.

Stage 4. Returning to purpose

At the last stage of 'Thinking Together', there must be a return to the overarching task. In our experience, this may often occur somewhat naturally since a mark of mentalized affect is that it moves the person from a more stuck position to a more flexible one. Mentalizing is indeed a 'theory of action'. What may occur at this stage may be likened to problem solving in which different options may be considered. It is again the responsibility of the worker's colleague to hold the AMBIT worker to the task implicit in this stage. The effort towards defining clear practical actions is needed and in this respect it is helpful to remember the 'START' criteria around any planned task. The five aspects of START are:

- Space (where is the space allocated for this work?)
- Time (how much time is allocated for this work?)
- Authority (who has authority?)
- Responsibility (who has responsibility?)
- Task (what actions need to be done?).

All 'Thinking Together' has a task that relates back to the search for some kind of product (a decision, an intervention, an understanding) that offers the promise of benefit for the client/family, and which will not harm them. The previous stages in this exercise represent a deliberate suspension of this task focus, to enable what we refer to as 'the curious exploratory play of ideas'.

If a decision cannot be made, or an understanding is not reached, then the practitioners may decide on further steps to enable this to move forward. This may involve thinking about who else might be required to advance the management of this problem. In extremis, the only plan that can be developed may carry things forward for just the next hour, for instance, and may involve emergency procedures or services. In less pressing situations, the AMBIT worker may need to resort to other formal supervisory structures such as the next (usually weekly) team meeting.

Mentalizing the network

One of the core features of AMBIT is the practitioner's stance of *taking responsibility for integration* (see above, pp. 171–172). Flowing from this is the specific application of this principle in regard to the wider network that surrounds the young person and their family.

AMBIT does not start from the rational position that all agencies working around a young person will easily be able to agree and work around a common purpose. It starts from a rather different position, i.e. that it is highly likely that the network of agencies (e.g. the police, mental health services, social care, schools and housing) involved in hard-to-reach young people have very different responsibilities towards the young person and that practitioners in these agencies often have very strong and different beliefs about what needs to be done. Our common experience is that it is often difficult to collaborate effectively with other agencies and that this is not to do with the unhelpful intentions of individual practitioners. The fact that difficulties in inter-agency working are often explained in terms of the intentions of others led us to consider the role of non-mentalizing in inter-agency work. In this way, we consider that it may be more productive to start from an assumption that all agencies and their practitioners will see things differently (i.e. in a non-integrated way) and will have different intentions with respect to the young person. What is needed is a method of exploring these differences without creating further blame.

The fundamental assumption we make is that network differences and conflicts should be anticipated as common and not be seen as an indication that people in the network around the young person are somehow 'getting it wrong'. This is crucial as it moves towards a more mentalized understanding of the complexities of multi-professional and multi-agency working. Because of the pervasiveness of the problems of this group (and, frequently, associated risks), the number of different professionals involved in these cases tends to multiply. However, clinical experience suggests that this 'team around the child' may experience difficulties in working together with this hard-to-reach group.

Because of this, the AMBIT practitioner is expected to pay close attention to the wider network around the young person and the family. For this population of young people, the network around the young person may consist of agencies which (even more than in other areas of child and adolescent mental health services, CAMHS) all see themselves as primary in relation to the young person. This may include the police, the local youth offending service, the young person's school or college, the local authority, and the local CAMHS. With this typical array of agencies, AMBIT adopts a position that actively anticipates the likelihood of conflict and contradiction between agencies or professionals, recognizing this as an inevitable aspect of their best efforts to provide services for the young person. In contrast to much of the literature on integrated practice (which tends to assume a commonality of purpose between different agencies), AMBIT proposes that a context of 'dis-integration' is extremely likely with this population of young people.

The 'dis-integration grid' is the basis of a simple brief exercise which can help AMBIT workers to make sense of the network around the young person. The worker can do this without using a proper form and can draw up a grid on a blank piece of paper at any time even during a multi-agency meeting if this is felt useful. An example of a dis-integration grid is shown in Figure 9.3.

The grid (designed as a tool to be deployed 'on the back of an envelope') simply invites the practitioner to map out the network around the young person by naming the key people in the network and then considering three questions about each of them in turn (the network should include a parent/

Levels	Worker	Young person	Parent(s)	Other services (add as required)
Conceptual What's the problem?				
Pragmatics What might help?				
System Whose responsibility is it to help?				

Figure 9.3 Dis-integration grid – connecting conversations. Copyright © Peter Fuggle and Dickon Bevington, Anna Freud Centre

carer). The task is to consider these three questions from the perspective of the other key people in the network. So, from each person's perspective, what is their belief as to:

1 Why is this problem happening?
2 What is likely to help?
3 Who should do this?

The questions are deliberately phrased to try to identify basic beliefs (in the realms of conceptual, pragmatic and systems thinking, where dis-integrations most frequently arise) rather than complicated, finely argued ideas. For example, a head of year in a school may believe that the young person's aggressive behaviour in school is due to the parent having no control at home. The perception is that the parent should take more authority at home and that it is her fault that she doesn't do this. In this way, the parent is seen as having the competence and authority to make the problem go away. Such a view may be completely different from her psychiatrist who is treating her for depression.

The idea of the grid is to map out the AMBIT worker's perceived beliefs of the key practitioners in the network. It is not intended that the AMBIT worker needs to know unambiguously what these are. The evidence for such beliefs may be based on detailed knowledge or on as little as third-party inter-agency gossip. The purpose of completing the dis-integration grid is to enable the AMBIT practitioner to mentalize (i.e. consider the behaviour of others with respect to intentional mental states) the young person's network and map out the differences and similarities in these perceptions, and in particular to identify if there are significant 'breaks' in the network, where different parts are pulling in opposing directions.

The aim here is to try to identify specific actions (what we might call 'connecting conversations') within a complex network that would aim to address some aspects of the dis-integration indicated from the grid. The question that we then invite the AMBIT worker to consider is: 'What conversations would be helpful to take place between whom in order for the network to work more effectively?' The intention here is not to try to fix the whole network, as this can often feel daunting and impossible, but to try to enable the AMBIT worker to take on specific tasks to enable the network to function in a more integrated way.

It needs to be emphasized that this is not just about improving coordination between agencies. The dis-integration grid does not address coordination but aims to encourage the AMBIT worker to become curious about the intentions and beliefs of others in the network. The rationale for this is that it may be very helpful to have discussions between network members about their different beliefs about what has caused the problem, as lack of coordination may be related to very different views about what needs to be done. This is a very different level of inter-agency dialogue than just coordinating different inputs.

Manualizing the practice

As described above, AMBIT is a manualized intervention, although the method of manualizing practice is different from manuals used in most treatment trials. In line with other manuals, the aim is to provide guidance on good practice for AMBIT workers around specific interventions or types of problems. For example, if an AMBIT worker wanted to be reminded of the basic steps in motivational interviewing, he could access this easily from the manual. Embedded video clips offer role plays that model therapeutic techniques and, increasingly, training modules are being added to this resource so as to reduce the cost of formal training.

As a wiki the AMBIT manual has a second purpose, which is to enable teams to reflect on *and to refine and document their own local practice*, considering what expertise they apply in implementing this material in response to the very specific demands of the local ecology. The intention is that teams may perform this 'self-manualization' as part of their routine team meetings or as part of their training and governance activities. In addition, AMBIT teams are encouraged to jointly develop their own protocols of good practice in relation to specific practice issues that may arise.

For example, a team may be working with young people who are very involved in gangs. The problem may be what to do if faced with young people who express a wish to leave a gang. There are no randomized controlled trials (RCTs) demonstrating unambiguously effective techniques in enabling young people to move away from gang membership. The team is likely to discuss this and develop ideas about good practice around this issue. This is then directly added into the manual and linked to other parts of the manual that are concerned with managing risk. In our opinion, the importance of this process with respect to mentalization is that the process of active manualization of good practice requires a staff team to consider many aspects of the issue, which promotes a mentalizing stance. As with 'Thinking Together' (see pp. 176–180) the aim is to encourage teams to move away from unstructured team discussion to boundaried discussions which facilitate more thinking.

Contrary to some expectations, using a web-based manual is easy and straightforward and can be achieved within the usual parameters of team working. The specific technology that supports this is a novel wiki technology, known as TiddlyWiki (www.tiddlywiki.com) and the AMBIT manual and its local variants can be found via the signposting site (www.tiddlymanuals.com). The AMBIT manual is supported by a rich online environment called TiddlySpace which allows multiple teams to integrate their own locally authored material independently around a shared common core – creating a *co-constructed manual* from centrally curated, and (ultimately we hope) 'evidence-based practice', and locally curated 'practice-based evidence'. The longer term aspiration is that over time teams in separate regions may have the potential to compare good practice ideas about common problems through comparing the differences and similarities of their specific manuals, and that best practice may be easily shared between teams. The AMBIT manual is open sourced, is freely downloadable and may be freely shared and adapted under the terms of its Creative Commons license.

Concusion

The application of mentalization-based approaches to the problems of highly socially excluded young people is still at an early stage. We have been encouraged by practitioners' responses to the training which we have delivered as this has tended to confirm its relevance and accessibility, but we are aware that systematic outcomes evaluation is essential as part of this early development work. Over the next two years, we have been funded to develop an AMBIT training programme for voluntary sector services working with the hard-to-reach client group and anticipate that this will enable us to further refine and evaluate the key components of the model described in this chapter.

For us, the value of mentalization as a core concept and practice in both work with young people and in team practice has been supported by its acceptability and accessibility to staff who have been trained in a wide range of models of practice, including those who may be somewhat distrustful of therapy models in general. Its particular value seems to be in asserting that the experience of high anxiety is a feature of working with multiply troubled young people and that this will inevitably compromise the practitioner's capacity to think about the young person's needs and situation. This common sense observation has been a powerful validation of practitioner experience and, at its best, enables practitioners to retain a sense of their own potential to facilitate positive change.

Acknowledgements

The work of the AMBIT team at the Anna Freud Centre, London, is generously supported by grants from Comic Relief, the City Bridge Trust and the Wentworth-Stanley Trust. We would like to thank them for the valuable support they have given us, which has made this work possible.

References

Addis, M. E., & Krasnow, A. D. (2000). A national survey of practicing psychologists' attitudes toward psychotherapy treatment manuals. *Journal of Consulting and Clinical Psychology*, 68(2), 331–339.

Fonagy, P., and Target, M. (2005). Bridging the transmission gap: An end to an important mystery of attachment research? *Attachment & Human Development*, 7(3), 333–343.

Fonagy, P., Gergely, G., Jurist, E. L., & Target, M. (2004). *Affect regulation, mentalization, and the development of the self.* New York: Other Press.

Henggeler, S. W., & Borduin, C. M. (1990). Treatment of delinquent behavior. In S. W. Henggeler & C. M. Borduin (Eds.), *Family therapy and beyond: A multisystemic approach to treating the behavior problems of children and adolescents* (pp. 219–245). Pacific Grove, CA: Brooks/Cole.

Henggeler, S. W., Rowland, M. D., Halliday-Boykins, C., Sheidow, A. J., Ward, D. M., Randall, J., *et al.* (2003). One year follow-up of multisystemic therapy as an alternative to the hospitalization of youths in psychiatric crisis. *Journal of the American Academy of Child and Adolescent Psychiatry*, 42(5), 543–551.

Hogue, A., Dauber, S., Samuolis, J., & Liddle, H. A. (2006). Treatment techniques and outcomes in multidimensional family therapy for adolescent behavior problems. *Journal of Family Psychology*, 20(4), 535–543.

Kessler, R. C., McLaughlin, K. A., Greif Green, J., Gruber, M., Sampson, N., Zaslavsky, A., *et al.* (2010). Childhood adversities and adult psychopathology in the WHO World Mental Health Survey. *British Journal of Psychiatry*, 197, 378–385.

Kipling, R. (1910). 'If'. *Collected poems of Rudyard Kipling*. Ware: Wordsworth Editions, 2001.

Liddle, H. A., Dakof, G. A., Parker, K., Diamond, G. S., Barrett, K., & Tejeda, M. (2001). Multidimensional family therapy for adolescent drug abuse: Results of a randomized clinical trial. *American Journal of Drug and Alcohol Abuse*, 27(4), 651–688.

Littell, J. H., Popa, M., & Forsythe, B. (2005). Multisystemic therapy for social, emotional, and behavioural problems in youth aged 10–17. *Cochrane Database of Systematic Reviews*, 4.

Swenson, C. C., Schaeffer, C. M., Henggeler, S. W., Faldowski, R., & Mayhew, A. M. (2010). Multisystemic therapy for child abuse and neglect: A randomized effectiveness trial. *Journal of Family Psychology*, 24(4), 497–507.

Chapter 10

A developmental approach to mentalizing communities through the Peaceful Schools experiment[1]

Stuart W. Twemlow, Peter Fonagy and Frank C. Sacco

Introduction

Applying attachment theory and mentalization concepts to complex social systems is an innovative use of these ideas. This chapter contrasts a social systems approach to school bullying and violence with a mentalization approach to the same problem and then attempts a synthesis of the two. We then summarize the findings of a test of these ideas in a randomized controlled trial (RCT) involving several schools and over 3000 children. Our goal in this chapter is to examine whether the serious contemporary problem of bullying and interpersonal violence in schools can be approached using a focus on the relationships between the members of the social system as a whole, rather than the more traditional strategy seen in prevention studies, i.e. that of identifying disturbed and at risk children and separating them from the social system for special attention.

A problem child as a symptom of a pathological social system

Let us begin with a vignette composed of details culled from several stories of everyday teaching disruptions by two middle-school teachers, who have been teaching for many years in a Midwestern school, in a low income area, in a mid-sized city in the US. The school has close to 2000 students and security guards guard its entryways. Violence is not uncommon in this school, including serious violence resulting in injury. The teachers in the school are divided into teams, each with a team leader, including one of the authors of this vignette. Each team is tasked with coordinating efforts to maintain a peaceful and productive classroom learning environment and curriculum.

1 Twemlow, S., Fonagy, P., & Sacco, F. (2005). A developmental approach to mentalizing communities: I The peaceful schools experiment. *Bulletin of the Menninger Clinic*, 69(4), 265–281. Reprinted with permission of Guilford Press.

The climate in this school is tense; teachers report often feeling frightened for their safety and desperate for support from the administration due to ongoing harassment from parents and children. They often do not feel they have the necessary social skills and psychological knowledge to cope with the children, many of whom they see as seriously disturbed, and frequently request that the children be separated from their peer group into special classrooms or referred for treatment.

The student at the center of our vignette, whom we shall call Billy, a slightly overweight round-faced 11-year-old, enters the classroom on a Monday morning, rushes to his desk, sits down with a loud commotion and yells out, 'I hate Mondays. School is such a waste of time.' The teacher, whom we shall call 'Ms. Jones', is allowing students to make up missing assignments during that particular class period. Billy has quite a few late Language Arts assignments to do. Billy makes it quite clear to Ms. Jones that Language Arts is the subject he hates the most and that he knows very well that he will not complete these assignments before the end of the period. Based on similar experiences, Ms. Jones knows that he plans to misbehave to cause conflict and avoid doing any work.

Initially, Ms. Jones tries to ignore Billy's initial comments and behaviour. She thinks to herself, 'Here we go again,' thus confirming her frustrations not only with Billy but with his mother, whom she felt was encouraging Billy's disruptive behaviour and constantly finding ways to criticize the school. Ms. Jones has become very frustrated with the situation, one that seemed to be escalating. She dreads the period that she has him because she knows that the help she requires is not available.

Billy's outburst is the culmination of many days of avoiding his work in numerous classes. When Ms. Jones mentions that she will call his mother, Billy becomes rude and indignant, adding that he couldn't care less because his mother thinks the school is 'stupid' anyway. Billy's comments only add to the mounting frustration that Ms. Jones feels about this particular school year, which in her view has seen a marked increase in complaints by displeased parents. She feels that the students realize they have the upper hand and can passively/aggressively manipulate their teachers because of their parents' and/or guardians' lack of faith in the public school system.

It seems to Ms. Jones that Billy has realized that he can get away with these daily disruptions because his mother, who is a single parent, allows it and is constantly threatening the school. When Ms. Jones has previously attempted to contact Billy's mother she has been treated with such disrespect that she now refuses to speak to the mother. All communication must go through the principal.

Every time Ms. Jones intervenes in an attempt to deter Billy's outbursts, his behaviour worsens. She asks him to sit down and keep quiet so that the other students may do their work without distraction, to stop making a nuisance of himself. With increasing emphasis she tells him to 'Stop making that noise!' to no avail. Finally, raising her voice she exclaims, 'Billy, just sit down! Now! And I mean it!' The escalation in behaviour that results from these failed interventions causes constant disruption to the class, leaving the remainder of the students unattended during various parts of the class period.

Unfortunately, when Ms. Jones finally refers Billy to the principal he is basically 'babysat' for the remainder of that period and is then sent to his next class. Ms. Jones feels that the principal refrains from more severe punishment in fear of reprisals to the school board by Billy's mother. Ms. Jones notes that Billy has had a history of difficulty with his peers since elementary school. He did not play collaboratively in elementary school and had trouble sharing playground equipment at recess. He seems always to have wanted to control and to dominate the mode of play. In basketball, he would pout if he was not elected captain of the team, and would make constant appeals, especially to male teachers to take his side.

By middle school it seems that his bullying behaviour made him feared and unpopular. He made an effort to associate with the popular peer group, but lacked the necessary social skills to carry off his role as a 'cool, popular kid'. His attempts at affiliation with the popular group did not give him the attention he seemed to need. He then tried to ally himself with the leader of the popular clique, as a sort of bodyguard, a role which was not always appreciated or appropriate. His classroom and peer relationship problems dominated his life, and of course led to a significant drop in his school grades.

Commentary from a mentalization perspective

From Ms. Jones' standpoint, Billy appears to be a boy capable of bullying teachers, and who through cunning manipulation of his mother and even the principal, achieves mafia-like protection from the system and an almost unlimited license to disrupt and maltreat teachers and students alike. While she is cognizant of his social failings, Ms. Jones has no genuine understanding of the reasons for his misbehaviour. Ms Jones assumes that Billy depicts with reasonable accuracy the beliefs and desires of those around him and has a developmentally adequate sense of his own psychic experiences. Thus it seems clear to her that his behaviour must be purposeful, aimed, for example, at avoiding work that he does not enjoy.

Ms. Jones does not blame Billy. She feels that the fault lies with Billy's mother, who communicates her attitude that the appropriate response to feeling bad in relation to the school is to attack it. In her attempt to find an explanation for Billy's behaviour, to contextualize his acts, Ms. Jones gropes towards exploring Billy's experiences of having been rejected by his peers. She sees his bullying as a solution he has found to achieve esteem, notwithstanding his brutishness and poor social skills. She sees a positively accelerating curve of bad behaviour feeding into poor performance in class, and further violence to protect Billy's basically flawed self-esteem.

Now let us take a second look at this scene, without some of the assumptions entailed by Ms. Jones' view of Billy as a basically rational person whose behaviour could be understood in terms of putative beliefs and desires. Ms. Jones, like all of us, tries to make sense of the actions of others as well as her own actions by reference to mental states. She does this spontaneously, intuitively and by and large not even consciously. Her mental attitude to Billy is qualitatively different from the way she might think about the physical world. The latter is understandable according to the laws of physics but at the core of her understanding of Billy is the unique assumption that Billy is a rational agent. Ms. Jones feels confident that she can 'divine' the beliefs that rational agent Billy ought to have held about his actions, his apparent goals and the context in which these occur. She even ventures to identify the desires underlying Billy's behaviour, his wish to avoid work. Basically as Daniel Dennett (1987) identified, she predicts that rational agent Billy will act to further his goals (to avoid any work) in the light of his belief that there are no substantial negative consequences to force alternative choices of action. Her model of Billy's behaviour seems to us reasonably accurate. It certainly appears to predict quite effectively what Billy goes on to do (that is, create further mayhem).

Beyond illustrating how we naturally and automatically form complex models of the behaviour of others in terms of their mental states, the vignette also illustrates the way mentalization interfaces with emotional life. Emotions relate to one's goals and desires. Ms. Jones' sense of frustration and hopelessness is rooted in her desire to modify Billy's behaviour and her belief that this is not a practically attainable goal.

Beliefs are representations of reality. There are no absolutes about beliefs in relation to particular experiences. Mentalization is by definition inexact. The mind is opaque. We have to share internal experiences with others to make them meaningful. Ms. Jones does not know that Billy is disrupting the class with the sole purpose of avoiding work, supported by the belief that he can get away with it. Recognizing the inherent uncertainty of mental states, offers us remarkable freedom to speculate about the nature of actions, to consider alternative perspectives and find an infinite variety of meanings behind behaviour.

Feeling the weight of the responsibility for the entire class, Ms. Jones does not give Billy the benefit of the doubt. She really does not know that Billy's exclamation 'I hate Mondays' is really borne of his desire to create turmoil motivated by his wish to avoid unpleasant work. Thus, Ms. Jones does not know that Billy's mother screamed at him before he left home, to get out of the house, to go to school, to leave her alone, adding for good measure, that she wished Billy 'had never been born'.

Billy's provocative (aggressive) behaviour driven by the emotional arousal gives rise to anxiety in Ms. Jones in relation to her responsibilities to the other students in the class. This prevents her from exploring possible alternative wishes behind Billy's behaviour. It never occurred to her to ask him what the matter was. Her reaction was to inhibit mentalization, to simplify matters and assume immediately that the past was repeating in the present. 'Here we go again', she said to herself without thinking of the specific instance. Billy gives only the faintest of indications of the nature of the turmoil he feels. When threatened with his mother's involvement, he expresses little apparent concern. He knows that for his mother the school is a convenient place to park Billy and that her overriding concern is not that he should have an education but that he should not be at home 'under her feet'.

But Ms. Jones' anxieties, which undermine her capacity to envision mental states, go beyond the interaction with Billy. Her failure to consider alternative accounts for Billy's behaviour may be linked to the threat that she experiences in relation to Billy's mother and all the other mothers and fathers who aggressively manipulate teachers and make thinking about beliefs and desires, thoughts and feelings well-nigh impossible. Ms Jones protects herself by refusing to have contact with Billy's mother; but at the same time she deprives herself of the opportunity to think about her and about what it could be like for an 11-year-old, far less well protected than she, to be the butt of this person's raging temper.

Unlike Ms. Jones, Billy does not have the opportunity to route all communications with his mother 'via the principal'. Perhaps at the beginning of the class when he made the commotion he was still feeling the impact of his mother's vitriolic onslaught and was not fully aware of the impact his behaviour was having on others but was simply trying to make himself feel better – not as Ms. Jones assumed to create an upheaval but to conceal his inadequacy. Contrary to Ms. Jones' belief, far from being able to manipulate the behaviour of his peers through creating distraction, Billy, with a limited capacity to mentalize, and being very afraid, is neither able to see their minds clearly nor anticipate their behaviour on the basis of their mental states, but instead makes sense of them on the basis of concrete behaviours.

He experiences the rebuke as an assault from yet another hostile mind which simply confirms his need to shut off, to make a noise, to disrupt, to protect himself from what is unbearably painful. Unable to tolerate hostile cognitions about him, he shuts out the entire person whose mind generates ideas that he experiences as malevolent. Ms. Jones, in feeling that she is not being listened to, naturally increases her wish to control and becomes increasingly physical in her manner of wanting to control Billy's behaviour. Were she able to reflect at this stage, she would recognize that her attitude simply pushes Billy further along in a non-mentalizing direction. And thus the classroom drama continues along its predictable path of emphasizing physical control (bullying), as opposed to influence through exploring and modifying feelings and ideas.

Looking at Billy as an agent whose rationality is limited by his impoverished ability to mentalize, particularly at times when he feels upset or anxious, helps us have a somewhat different appreciation of not only his current behaviour but also his history. Billy's father is absent, not there to protect him from his mother, but also not there to help Billy see his situation from an alternative standpoint. Billy has neither older siblings nor a father present to perform this task. In fact none of the adult figures around him assist him with the terror he sometimes feels around the mother that he also critically depends upon. Even the school principal appears to be frightened of his mother and so does Ms. Jones, although neither of these well-intentioned people recognizes that their reaction of acquiescence to Billy's mother further exaggerates Billy's fear of her. They don't think of it – not because they are unthinking people – but because they have specific difficulty in thinking about thoughts and feelings in relation to Billy.

Billy so clearly appears to lack the capacity to be attuned with his peers, reacting to them in ways that they find disturbing, even at times when he was overanxious to please. He would then repeatedly do the wrong thing; making himself an object of ridicule. He inadequately defends against this state which all of us would find almost unbearable by creating a position for himself through coercion and sometimes cruelty. No one notices that these instances of cruelty are almost invariably linked to moments where he feels profoundly humiliated by those around him. No one notices because the kind of physicalistic strategies that he uses to control the minds of those around him are precisely what exclude the possibility of mentalization. Billy has created a system around him, which increasingly responds solely to physical threats rather than reason.

Billy is a bodyguard and as such commands respect rather than ridicule. Most of his peers see him as overconfident. If asked, they would say that Billy thinks he is great, a cool kid. Few notice how his determination to stay on top is driven by desperation. Unlike most other boys Billy is not able to set aside social criticism as something which is just one person's perspective. He feels it as if it was directly destroying him. Functioning in a physical equivalence mode, humiliation and shame could destroy him totally because he experiences such thoughts directly almost as if they could have a physical impact. Of course, neither his peers, nor his teacher or the principal can truly appreciate what this feels like.

So, how can we help Billy? Or Ms. Jones in her struggle with him? It would be impractical to try to explain the intricate communication patterns we have outlined above. If we had asked Ms. Jones to consider even a tiny proportion of these elaborations, she would be far too busy having to cope with an entire class. Would Billy benefit from individual therapy?

Experience shows that boys like Billy respond poorly to such efforts, however skilled, if not occurring in the context of concurrent family and social interventions. Therefore we feel that disrupting the vicious cycle that Billy finds himself in should also be undertaken in Billy's school and class. Further, it may be best, given Billy's sensitivity to humiliation, if the intervention does not directly concern Billy at all but rather the whole class.

It may seem like using a sledgehammer to crack a nut to modify the behaviour of the class rather than imposing consequences on Billy. Yet if we take a broader view we can see that it is not just Billy but all those interacting with him who have difficulty in considering thoughts and feelings. The problems may originate in Billy but Ms. Jones, normally a sensitive and caring person, finds herself reacting to Billy by shouting and bullying. Her reactions in turn paralyse the other children to a point where there is little expectation on anyone's part that thinking about what is going on could achieve more than imposing physical consequences. The procedure in the context of our programme would have been for Ms. Jones to stop the class immediately after Billy started creating a commotion and mark some space for reflection on what was happening. Later in this chapter more specific details about the process are given in the section on Classroom Management (pp. 196–197).

Commentary from a social system–power dynamics perspective

The social systems perspective makes certain assumptions about the way social systems operate. Of particular importance in this application is the way in which Billy immediately forces everybody's attention to his problems, by coercive misery, provocation and contempt: 'School is a waste of time and you won't do anything till you deal with my problems!' Unwittingly, Ms. Jones has been dragged into the role of victim as Billy adopts the victimizer role. Billy has likely learnt this pattern by observing aggressiveness in the home. Power has achieved primitive control objectives for him, modelled by his parents and other family members. Ms. Jones is at the end of her tether with Billy and his mother, and demonstrates the incapacitating power of the victim's role by her impoverished and uncreative thoughts to herself; the 'here we go again' feeling, which creates a feeling of being defeated from the outset. Billy, although he may be crying out for help, has also unwittingly adopted a position of power that is facilitated and even enhanced by the submissiveness of the surrounding bystander system that cannot cope with him.

Research has shown that in serious aggression, submission encourages a controlling grandiose response by projective identification of disavowed self-representations into the victimizer (Twemlow, 1995a, 1995b). Thus, the victimizer becomes locked in a hateful 'dance', which decreases the capacity to think and increases the tendency to stereotype the other, all in an ambience that is not conducive to creative and constructive compromises. This school has literally run out of ideas about Billy!

From this perspective, Billy's fundamental problem is a systemic one. He is a pawn in a much larger social game, a game that involves his ever-changing role as bully and victim in the interchange with his social group, both of his teachers and of his peers. The victimized response of the authority system, especially the teachers who have to deal with him directly, and the audience of bystanders who occupy a variety of different roles, unwittingly aggravate the victimization. This enhances Billy's ability to control the system by his complaining (victim role), and his carping aggressiveness (bully role), thus reducing the probability that learning can occur for anybody in the school. If Billy's problems are to be contained and he is to become part of a creative and peaceful school-learning environment, the assumption is that these pathological roles have equal culpability and responsibility.

The energy or power of the system that positions Billy in the dominating role arise from the failure to deal with the power dynamic that keeps it going. This perspective depicts the bystander in a less obvious role, which nonetheless is a key, we feel, to normalizing the system. Bystanders, all of whom feel disempowered by the combined force of Billy and his mother, include all school personnel – administration, parents, teachers, volunteers, support staff and security personnel, as well as of course the students. Billy has heard that his mother feels that the school is stupid, so the mother has created here a folie à deux; she has become, like Billy, engaged in a power struggle with the school, attempting to control it to do her will.

In the position of the victim Ms. Jones is overwhelmed and discouraged and is now going to the principal for help, since she has realized most likely that her rage and helplessness is a reactive concrete repetition of Billy's role as victim. Thus the talion principle reigns in this school, with an accompanying mindset that tends to stereotype and oversimplify human relationships. Billy becomes an intolerable monster. People have become dehumanized part objects rather than whole individuals and the problem escalates.

The power struggle in the pathological social system has become even worse because the principal has also been disempowered, becoming an exaggerated babysitter for Billy, most likely conveying to Billy that he is in control of the principal, the teacher and the whole school. This constitutes an overwhelming burden for a child of 11 who is developmentally trying to contain aggression; he may be both exhilarated in a triumphant sense and terrified by such developmentally inappropriate power. The failure of the parental authorities to contain and hold his aggressiveness further escalates the problem, which he most likely acts out at home with more aggressiveness. Higher authorities then become the focus of attention when mother threatens to report the school to the school board. Billy's attempts to appeal to a higher authority, such as the principal, his mother and others can be viewed from one perspective as adaptive maneuvers. That is, the regressed quality of the thinking of those trapped in this spiralling aggression becomes oversimplified into a search for a helpful dominant hierarchy in which the more powerful can subdue and control the weak. In most human social systems there is no ultimate authority that can completely control a system, so with the philosophy in Billy's middle school the system has no option but to continue to flounder without direction.

In summary, all personnel in Billy's life have at different times adopted the roles of bully, victim and bystander even from one classroom period to another. The social systems–power dynamics perspective sees this as a dissociating process; the bully on behalf of the bystanding community dissociates the victim from the school community as 'not us'. In this instance Billy is the bully in terms of overt behaviour, but he is also the victim of a group process; the community bystander role can be described as an abdicating one. The abdicating bystander projects blame for problem children onto others, often those in the school system, such as teachers, administrators and school security personnel. From this vantage point any intervention in the school setting must focus on the transformation of the bystander into a committed community member. A successful intervention should promote recognition within the large school group of the dissociated elements represented by the victim Billy, as a scapegoat for a larger group problem to which each member of the group contributes as a bystander.

This dissociating process is a largely unconscious effort to deal with the anxiety felt by all in response to a dysfunctional, coercive and disconnected social system. Any remedy for this state of affairs requires a clear conceptualization of the group's task from a perspective that does not permit scapegoating, empowers bystanders into a helpful altruistic role and does not overemphasize the importance of therapeutic efforts with the victim or victimizer. The symptom, bullying, is not merely a problem to solve, but a dysfunctional solution or adaptation, which obscures a larger and more painful and meaningful problem, the dysfunctional social context.

The Peaceful Schools project: a mentalizing social system

In general, social systems which are incompatible with violence, are mentalizing social systems. This is because an individual is, from an evolutionary point of view, usually incapable of exercising interpersonal aggression in a context in which they successfully mentalize their victim, unless the social system has assigned the action as necessary aggression, e.g. attacking for the sake of food or protection (Fonagy, 2003). The difference between a violent and a non-violent community must then be the degree to which the implicit social conventions are structured to encourage all participants to be aware of the mental states of others of that group and to take these into account when forming rules and regulations and procedures for the system.

Is it possible to create a mentalizing social system with balanced power dynamics? In 1992, we began an experiment in schools, designed to test that hypothesis. The first seven years of the study involved piloting and refining interventions and the results of these efforts are reported in detail elsewhere (Twemlow, 2000; Twemlow *et al.*, 2001a, 2001b, 2002). The inciting incident was the attempted rape of a second grade girl by several second grade boys, in a school with the highest out of school suspension rate in the school district and the poorest academic performance on standardized achievement tests. After this phase, in which the school did very well, a randomized controlled trial was conducted involving nine elementary (K-5) schools and over 3600 students.

The basis of the approach encouraged the creation of a philosophy rather than a programme. In doing so the reflective component of mentalizing is encouraged since everyone involved participates in the process and does not merely follow a dehumanized research protocol. Understanding how the system works from the mentalizing power dynamics perspective allows the individual teachers and students to create innovative ways of moulding that social climate in the school. The components of the programme philosophy included the following:

1. Positive climate campaigns

These campaigns use counsellor-led discussions, posters, magnets, bookmarks and other devices to encourage a shift in language and thinking of all students and personnel in the school. These language tools help identify and resolve problems that develop when coercive power dynamics dominate the school environment. For example, children help each other resolve issues without adult participation. Such effects are observed as they share playground equipment peacefully and do not push and jostle in the lunch line. This creates a context in which no participant can experience the situation without awareness of the mental state of the other and indeed without self awareness; instead, the focus is on the relationship between bully, victim and bystander, which implicitly creates a demand on the child, the teacher and other staff to consider this interpersonal situation from a mentalizing perspective.

2. Classroom management (discipline plan)

This approach assists teachers' efforts at discipline by focusing on correcting root problems, instead of punishing and criticizing behaviours. A behaviour problem in a single child is conceptualized as a problem for the whole class who participate in bully, victim or bystander roles. Scapegoating is reduced and insight into the meaning of the behaviour becomes paramount. From this new perspective, a child's disruptive behaviour is seen as an attempt to locate a valid social role within the group. At the point of disruption, the teacher would stop teaching and assign bully, victim and bystander roles during class discussion. The bully being the child, the victim being the teacher and the bystanders would be the rest of the classroom, who may have laughed at the teacher's response to the disruptive student.

If such a child repeatedly offends, the class would collectively fill out a power struggle referral alert. That is every student would participate in determining and defining the bullying, victim and bystander behaviour according to a standardized form. At a later point the children involved and sometimes even the parents of the child would be seen by the school counsellor or social worker for a further understanding of the event. This process and other aspects of the Peaceful Schools approach are presented to parents in regular workshops entitled 'Six People, One Bathroom', where the opportunity is also taken to help teach the approach to parents to use in resolving their power issues in the home situation and to mentalize their children.

The child with a propensity to act violently is encouraged by this approach to develop a mental life representation of his experiences and adapt to it in a non-persecutory way. The essential component of this approach is that children do not experience themselves as having been punished, which would inhibit, rather than facilitate mentalization. So the environment becomes conducive to thinking within the context of a counselling relationship that encourages mentalization. The purpose is to encourage the child to think about the perspective of others, including his or her parents as well as teachers and principals. Experience suggests that teachers who invoke punishment less frequently in response to classroom behaviours show classrooms with better academic performance and fewer disciplinary referrals.

3. Peer and adult mentorship

Mentorship approaches are attempts to mirror outside the classroom what the classroom management plan does in the classroom. That is to get everybody in the school system to understand the violent interaction, and to see if there is a way to resolve the problem collaboratively and without blame. Male mentors seem particularly helpful on the playground where much childhood aggression comes out. The most effective male mentors are rather relaxed older men of any race, often retired, non-competitive, who have children and grandchildren of their own. One particularly skilled mentor cleverly used magic tricks to distract children. He would make himself a buffer – for example, 'Why don't you go first on the climbing frame and I will try and catch each of you'. Thus the fight becomes a game with him as the referee.

Looking at mentoring from a mentalizing perspective requires the point of view of the 'third' (Ogden, 1994). Ogden considers that this co-created 'third', the melded inter-subjectivities, allows the analyst to attend and think clearly about the patient. For example, the mentalizing action of the mentor and his game creates a transitional space by this distraction in which the participants, the bully, the victim and the bystander, start thinking in this space, thus allowing disruptive affect to settle, with a spontaneity essential for mentalizing, and with the hope that this modelling eventually will be internalized by the children, so that the model relationship in the mind of the children, creates the helpful 'third' in the abstract.

4. The gentle warrior physical education programme

This approach satisfies the physical education requirements in most school systems, using a combination of role playing, relaxation and defensive martial arts techniques. The approach helps children protect themselves and others with non-aggressive physical and cognitive strategies. For example, occupying bully, victim and bystander roles provides students with alternatives to fighting and a mentalized grasp of the mindset of different roles. Learning ways to physically defend oneself, when being grabbed, pushed or shoved, combined with classroom discussion, teaches personal self-control as well as respect and helpfulness towards others. These confidence-building skills support an essential component of the capacity to mentalize, which is to allow children to feel confident enough and safe enough to be able to think. If a child is too frightened, the capacity to think is paralysed and the victim mindset is adopted.

5. Reflection time

Adler (1958) pointed out that a natural social group has no right to exclude any member, or conversely, that every member of the group has a right to belong. From his point of view, narcissistic injury represented by bully, victim and some bystander reactions are attempts by the child to regain entry into a social group and to be accepted by that social group. Although teachers may see the Peaceful Schools programme as training the child, the real aim is that the teachers actively become involved in mentalizing the child via the process of training. The serious problem of teachers who bully and are bullied by students and parents (Twemlow *et al.*, 2004; Twemlow & Fonagy, 2005) is one example of how important the mentalizing teacher becomes to this process. So the system through its members becomes more psychologically aware and eventually the rules, regulations and policy of the system will embody mentalizing principles.

Reflection time is one such method to encourage mentalizing in teachers and students. This period of ten minutes or so at the end of each day is when the classroom engages in a discussion of the day's activities from the point of view of bully, victim and bystander behaviour, and after discussing this behaviour make a decision about whether to display a banner outside the classroom indicating that the class has had a good day. Teachers note that the children are rather critical of themselves and do not put up the banner as much as the teachers might. Thus, mentalizing children are capable of being self-critical without a drop in self-esteem. In many ways the subject of the reflection matters less than that the reflection is taking place.

Results of the Peaceful School projects

The complex structured methodology and analytic strategy for this project is described in detail elsewhere (Fonagy *et al.*, 2005, 2009). In summary, a traditional school psychiatric consultation (SPC) was compared to an intervention based on a mentalizing and power dynamics systems approach as described in the body of this chapter (creating a peaceful school learning environment, CAPSLE), and a treatment as usual (TAU) condition in which schools had been promised whichever was the more successful of the other two interventions in return for collecting data. The study was a cluster level randomized controlled trial with stratified restricted allocation. Efficacy was assessed after two years of active intervention and effectiveness after one year of minimal input maintenance intervention.

Nine elementary schools with 1345 third to fifth graders (8- to 11-year-olds) provided data for the trial, which was conducted in a medium sized Midwestern city in the USA. Approximately 3600 children were exposed to the interventions. The outcome of the interventions were measured with peer and self-reports of bullying and victimization, peer reports of aggressive and helpful bystanding, self-reports of empathy towards victims of bullying, self-reports of belief that aggression is legitimate and classroom and behavioural observation of disruptive and off-task behaviour.

Longitudinal research has shown that there is usually an increase in levels of peer-reported aggression between third and fifth grade. However, analysis of the data suggested that CAPSLE moderated the developmental trend of increasing peer-reported victimization ($p < .01$), aggression ($p < .05$), self-reported aggression ($p < .05$) and aggressive bystanding ($p < .05$), compared to TAU schools. CAPSLE also moderated a decline in empathy and an increase in the percent of children victimized compared to SPC ($p < .01$) and TAU conditions ($p < .01$).

Results for self-reported victimization, helpful bystanding, and beliefs in the legitimacy of aggression did not suggest significantly different changes among the study conditions over time. CAPSLE produced a significant decrease in off-task ($p < .001$) and disruptive classroom behaviours ($p < .01$), while behavioural change was not observed in SPC and TAU schools. Superiority with respect to TAU for victimization ($p < .05$), aggression ($p < .01$), and helpful ($p < .05$) and aggressive bystanding ($p < .01$) were maintained in the follow-up year.

The results of this study, which are reported more fully in Fonagy *et al.* (2009) suggest that a teacher-implemented school-wide intervention that does not focus on disturbed children substantially reduced aggression and improved classroom behaviour. The major conclusion was that this programme philosophy was effective in reducing children's experiences of aggressiveness and victimization, even though it did not focus at all on the identified problem children, i.e. the bully and victim and that children did become more involved in helping to reduce aggressiveness as suggested by the increasing engagement of Peaceful Schools' children in helpful bystanding behaviours.

Follow-up of children into middle school suggests maintained academic performance of children exposed to the Peaceful Schools philosophy for more than two years, even if placed in a non-peaceful school.

Conclusion

In this chapter we have attempted to synthesize a theoretical/philosophical perspective on mentalizing and power dynamics as a type of attachment pattern between individuals that is essential to how social systems, like schools operate, with experimental data to support that viewpoint. The larger question of whether a community can reflect the mentalizing power-dynamics perspective in the way it organizes itself remains unanswered. Our feeling is that for communities to reflect the high quality of life demanded by citizens in an open democracy, such changes in how the system as a whole operates must occur.

Acknowledgements

We would like to thank Megan and Brad Culver, who provided the case vignette and discussed with us their rewarding but stressful experiences teaching in US Public Schools. This research was supported by Foundation grants to Child & Family Program, Menninger Dept. Psychiatry, Baylor College Medicine, Houston, TX. This chapter is a revised and edited version of a paper published in the *Bulletin of the Menninger Clinic*, 2005, 69(4), 265–281.

References

Adler, A. (1958). *What life should mean to you.* New York: Putnam Capricorn Books.
Dennett, D. (1987). *The intentional stance.* Cambridge, MA: MIT Press.

Fonagy, P. (2003). Towards a developmental understanding of violence. *British Journal of Psychiatry*, 183, 190–192.

Fonagy, P., Twemlow, S. W., Vernberg, E., Sacco, F. C., & Little, T. D. (2005). Creating a peaceful school learning environment: Impact of an antibullying program on educational attainment in elementary schools, *Medical Science Monitor*, 11(7), 317–325.

Fonagy P., Twemlow S., Vernberg, E., Mize, J., Dill, E., Little, T., *et al.* (2009). Randomized controlled trial of a child-focused psychiatric consultation and a school systems-focused intervention to reduce aggression. *Journal of Child Psychology and Psychiatry*, 50(5), 607–616.

Ogden, T. (1994). *Subjects of analysis*. Lanham, MD: Jason Aronson.

Twemlow, S. W. (1995a). The psychoanalytical foundations of a dialectical approach to the victim/victimizer relationship. *The Journal of the American Academy of Psychoanalysis*, 23(4), 545–561.

Twemlow, S. W. (1995b). Traumatic object relations configurations seen in victim/victimizer relationships. *The Journal of the American Academy of Psychoanalysis*, 23(4), 563–580.

Twemlow, S. W. (2000). The roots of violence: Converging psychoanalytic explanatory models for power struggles and violence in school. *Psychoanalytic Quarterly*, 69(4), 741–785.

Twemlow, S. W., Fonagy, P., Sacco, F. C., Gies, M., Evans, R., & Ewbank, R. (2001a). Creating a peaceful school learning environment: A controlled study of an elementary school intervention to reduce violence. *American Journal of Psychiatry*, 158(5), 808–810.

Twemlow, S. W., Fonagy, P., & Sacco, F. C. (2001b). An innovative psychodynamically influenced intervention to reduce school violence. *Journal of the American Academy of Child and Adolescent Psychiatry*, 40(3), 377–379.

Twemlow, S. W., Fonagy, P., & Sacco, F. (2002). Feeling safe in school. *Smith College Studies in Social Work*, 72(2), 303–326.

Twemlow, S., Fonagy, P., & Sacco, F. (2004). The role of the bystander in the social architecture of bullying and violence in schools and communities. *Annals of New York Academy of Sciences*, 1036, 215–232.

Twemlow, S. W., & Fonagy, P. (2005). A note on teachers who bully students in schools with differing levels of behavioral problems. *American Journal of Psychiatry*, 162(12), 2387–2389.

Chapter 11

'Thoughts in Mind'

Promoting mentalizing communities for children

Poul Lundgaard Bak

Introduction

The development of the 'Thoughts in Mind' project

Mentalizing can be defined as the ability to 'read' other people's thoughts and feelings and to reflect upon one's own thoughts and feelings. As earlier chapters have outlined in more detail, the ability to mentalize develops gradually through childhood, depending greatly on the establishment of secure relationships with parents, other adults and friends. Research also suggests that mentalization is an important factor behind coping, mental health and behaviour. Hence, the development of mentalizing communities is of great interest both to the individual and to future society.

Finding creative ways to bring an awareness of the importance of mentalizing to those working with – and caring for – children is a priority. Recent research indicates that mentalization can be supported by school education programmes (see Twemlow *et al.*, Chapter 10). The Danish Thoughts in Mind (TiM – in Danish *OmTanke projektet*) project was inspired by this research, but has somehow tried to go further in making mentalizing ideas as widely available as possible among those caring for children.

The TiM concepts and materials (including lecture and training plan for staff and parents) were developed and pilot tested between 2005 and 2009. The organizational setting of the project is the department for children and adolescents in Aarhus, the second largest city in Denmark. The department serves 60,000 children in schools and day-care centres. There are 15,000 employees in the organization (such as teachers, educators, etc.).

TiM was developed within this setting as a low-intensity, group-based programme for teachers, day-care staff and parents aimed at stimulating a mentalizing environment for children as an integral part of their daily life and activities. This can happen through questioning, storytelling, or plays – thereby empowering individuals and groups as well as increasing teacher and parent skills in their daily learning environment. The programme is designed for large-scale implementation in real community settings with limited resources. That the mentalizing capacity of parents is important for the mental health of their children is well known from attachment theory and research. The hypothesis in this project is that even minor changes in the adult mentalizing community around children can have significant impact on their mental health, simply because parents and teachers spend thousands of hours with their children. TiM can be considered as inspirational and practical 'knowledge vitamins' about thoughts, feelings and the brain for adults working with children and adolescents, and thus is a programme which aspires to stimulate a mentalizing community for children.

Basic TiM concepts as presented to parents and teachers

A crucial core of the TiM project is to translate scientific theory and knowledge about mentalization into practical knowledge at the children's own level (in narratives, images and metaphors) – with the purpose of giving inspiration to professionals and parents within a realistic time and resource framework, and stimulating reflections, conversations, practice, observations and plays around mentalization. For this purpose, a 70-page TiM booklet has been produced together with a small film and models for short lectures and courses. The lectures are designed to give the best possible appetizers, hopefully raising curiosity and a desire to dive deeper into the material and the understanding of oneself and others and to explore how mentalization unfolds in daily life and relations.

However, the TiM programme must be considered as a gateway to the world of mentalization and cannot be compared to a classic parent education or cognitive training programme with, for example, ten or more planned sessions, including lectures and rehearsals. It is a deliberate choice of the TiM project to experiment with this kind of low-cost intervention to see how far one can get with a carefully designed workshop aimed to inspire – or stimulate – a mentalizing stance within a community-based intervention. Even though we already have interesting stories from professionals and parents who use TiM techniques to help their children cope with challenges and conflicts in their life (see below, pp. 212–214), TiM is basically considered as a mental health education programme and not as a treatment. However, any family should also, of course, have full access to this kind of knowledge and information.

The following description reveals how the reader is introduced to the world of thoughts and feelings in the TiM booklet or workshop:

> Even though thoughts and feelings are extremely complicated events occurring within us, they are, at the same time, very common in that we experience them all the time.

> Thoughts and feelings are important and practical, they can be exciting and pleasant, and they can be difficult and unpleasant. Thoughts and feelings, whether strong or mild, have consequences, especially when they are expressed in actions.
>
> Obviously, it is more difficult to discover invisible events than visible ones in the world around us. Therefore, children gradually discover that things do occur inside their own heads and not in other people's heads when they are 3–5 years old. From that age, it is a voyage of discovery throughout life to understand and use one's thoughts and feelings as a means to bring joy and benefit to oneself and others.
>
> Obtaining new knowledge gives us further choices in life – just think what new technology has brought into our everyday life. We continuously acquire new knowledge about the brain and about thoughts and feelings, providing us with even more new options. This is not without interest considering that the brain is, after all, the most important 'computer' in our lives.
>
> This booklet contains simple and practical knowledge about thoughts, feelings and the brain as well as some short stories, games, and illustrations. Hopefully, the booklet can provide inspiration in everyday life – a kind of 'knowledge vitamins' about thoughts and feelings, health, and well-being.
>
> The booklet is also about mindreading – about reading your thoughts. And that is exactly the same process as when learning to read. With this booklet, you can begin to play with your child using the 'mindreading alphabet'. If the child finds this activity meaningful and fun and you practise it together, you help your child to decipher the 'mindreading code' and the door opens to a world of many possibilities – just like in the world of books.
>
> (Lundgaard Bak, 2009: 3–4)

The booklet then goes on to provide a set of narratives that aim to introduce basic concepts about thoughts and feelings to parents and teachers. It begins with presenting the fundamental idea that inside ourselves we have something we call 'I' (the self agent, as described by Fonagy *et al.*, 2002).

> The actual concept of this 'I' is very difficult to concretize – and it is a question we don't need to answer within this context. So far, it is enough for us to know that we have an 'I'. Just notice how often the word 'I' is used in conversations. The 'I' experiences the world by paying attention to things, that is by using a kind of invisible 'spotlight' to discover the world and get to know it. From the point of the 'I', the world consists of three levels inside each other:

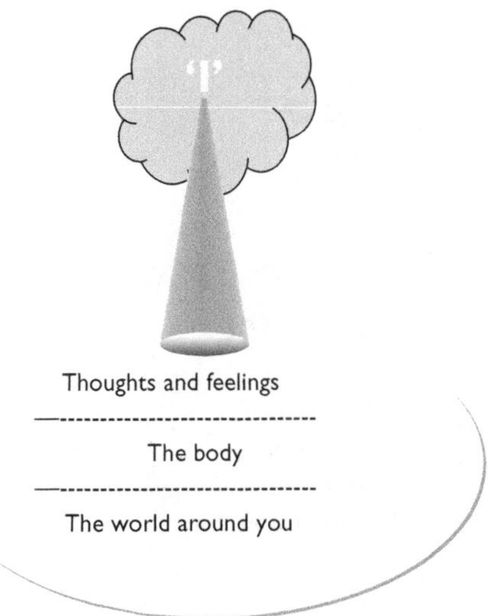

Figure 11.1 The levels of reality

- The world around you (people, nature, things) that you can see, hear, smell, touch and taste.
- The body – which you can feel.
- Thoughts and feelings which you experience inside yourself.

> The 'I' is quite like the spotlight on stage in a theatre. The spotlight highlights the most important thing on stage at a particular moment. Metaphorically speaking the 'I' is the lighting director, your attention is the spotlight, and the stage is your world. (See Figure 11.1.)

This little game illustrates the principle:

> You need an ordinary torch. Switch on the torch and hold it in one hand along the side of your head – just like a headlamp. Turn your head, so the light points at one particular point. Shift your gaze and focus your attention on this particular point. Maintain light, gaze, and attention on the point for a few seconds. Then turn your head, hand, torch, and attention to another point in the room and keep your light, gaze, and attention on this new point for a few seconds.
>
> It is your 'I' that controls the muscles of your head, your hand, the torch, the direction of the light, your eyes, sight and attention – and your 'I' experiences the object at exactly the same second as it is spotlighted in the centre of attention. So, at THIS very moment, YOU are the one that decides what you experience.
>
> (Lundgaard Bak, 2009: 8–10)

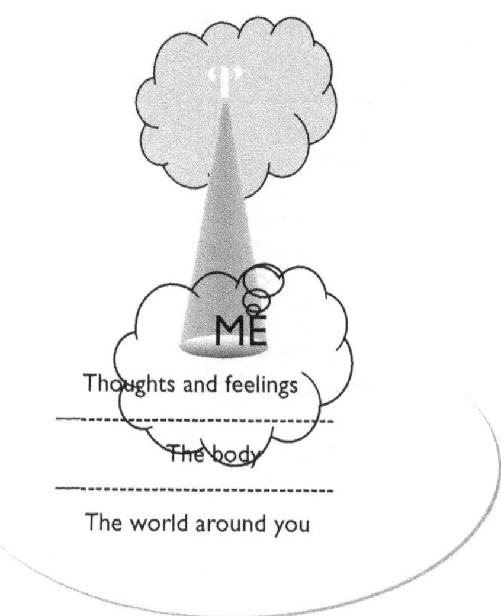

Figure 11.2 I and me

This game, which in the workshop we demonstrate using an actual torch, can also illustrate how the 'I' can turn its attention towards thoughts and feelings, experience thoughts and feelings, and shift its attention to other thoughts and feelings (see Figure 11.2). We aim to encourage those reading or hearing about this game to be playful and try out different things:

> Try to cut out different-sized 'thought bubbles' in different colours – symbolizing big and small thoughts in 'happy' and 'sad' colours. You can write in the 'thought bubbles' as well. Spread them out on a table, or hold them against the forehead as though they were thoughts inside your head.
>
> Use the torch as a 'spotlight' – your attention. The hand holding the torch symbolizes the 'I' that can focus/shed light on a thought – and shift focus to another thought.
>
> When the 'I' (the hand) holds 'tightly' onto the attention (the torch), it is like focusing on a certain thought. Play with the torch and shift focus from one thought to another. Hold the torch (and the attention inside your head) tightly and concentrate for a moment on a specific thought.
>
> From the very first moment in your life, you experience the world around you. Consequently you build up a thought model of the world inside your brain. Look at an object in front of you – and you will discover and experience the object simultaneously. Close your eyes – and you are able to imagine the same object even though you cannot

> see it. You now have a thought model of the object that you can experience.
>
> You also experience 'who you are'. It is your image of yourself – your identity. Your image of yourself is a pattern of thoughts and feelings which you have built up and now experience within yourself.
>
> (Lundgaard Bak, 2009: 13–14)

In the workshop and TiM materials we try to illustrate this way of thinking about 'who you are' by inviting people to use the paper 'thought bubbles' and a torch and to draw or write on one or more of the 'thought bubbles' how they perceive themselves and the kind of person they would like to become. We then encourage them to play around and move the 'spotlight' to who they want to be. We use games like this to illustrate how the 'I' can decide about thoughts and feelings in a split second – by shifting its focus of attention to what 'I' would like to think about – at this particular moment.

But we also invite participants to think about the fact that the 'I' does not always decide, that important events in the inner and outer world can attract its attention – even though the 'I' doesn't want them to. The 'I' can be frightened if something happens very suddenly, something which seems dangerous – with or without cause; the 'I' can feel quite ill if an unpleasant feeling overwhelms it; or the stomach or head can ache so badly that the 'I' cannot think about anything else at all. Once again, the drawing of attention can be illustrated by using the paper 'thought bubbles' and the torch:

> Imagine that one of the thought bubbles symbolizes an important (positive or negative) inner or outer event – and that this event is so important that it draws your attention 'like a magnet' – in a way that the spotlight/attention (the torch) is very close to the event (the thought bubble).
>
> This means that there is a lot of light and attention on whatever is important at this particular moment while all the other possible thoughts and feelings outside the light and attention are 'in the dark' – i.e. they don't exist when you are completely absorbed in something really important.
>
> Imagine it like being on stage in a theatre when the spotlight hits a small area on the stage, and everything else becomes 'invisible' because it is in the dark.
>
> So the 'I' keeps hold of one end of the attention, while events in the inner and outer world keep hold of the other end. In every single second throughout life, there is an ongoing game about who is in control of our attention – the 'I' or events in the outer and inner world.

> Your personal freedom concerns how you take part in deciding what goes on in your life. When YOU, often consciously, decide *what* you will think about *right NOW*, you are training your ability to control your thoughts and feelings – so *you* are in control of your own thoughts and feelings, and not vice versa. Life consists of many successive 'NOWS' . . . so there are many opportunities to practise this inner self control in a way that it becomes easier to remain focused and attentive when being in the company of others, as well as when meeting challenges, solving problems, and completing tasks.
>
> (Lundgaard Bak, 2009: 15–16)

In the TiM material, there are small stories illustrating the basic concepts. They are not real stories with figures and acts, but rather meta-narrative stories creating metaphoric frames for thoughts, feelings and mentalization in which the listener can fill in his or her own personal metaphors, thoughts, and feelings. It is well known that the experience of being able to cope with challenges in life events is extremely important for one's well-being and health. Most often coping is connected with challenges and events in the 'outside' world or in the body (illness and diseases). The purpose of the meta-narrative stories is to stimulate mental metaphors and strategies for coping inside one's own mind. Here is one of the stories:

The story of the House of Thoughts

> In a way, it can be said that our thoughts live inside our heads. Imagine that your thoughts live in a house with many rooms where you can wander around and discover them.
>
> When you discover thoughts, you are using the world's finest tool – your attention, which is a kind of spotlight. When you spotlight a thought, you 'discover' it. Attention can then be shifted and you discover another thought.
>
> The House of Thoughts has many rooms. Some exciting thoughts may live in one room, maybe some sad or angry thoughts live in another room, and yet in a third room happy and pleasant thoughts reside.
>
> In the House of Thoughts, thoughts can call on you if they want to be discovered. This can be exciting and really good, but it can be irritating as well – especially if annoying thoughts keep butting in and try to take over your attention *all the time*.
>
> If specific thoughts want to make you stay in their room all the time, they may prevent you from discovering all the thoughts in the other rooms.
>
> If you have sad or angry thoughts wanting you to retreat into *their* room all the time, you may end up believing that there aren't any

exciting or happy thoughts to be found anywhere, and this is not at all funny . . .

But this is not the case. All the happy and exciting thoughts are present, waiting in the other rooms of the House of Thoughts, waiting for you to discover them with your spotlight.

The House of Thoughts is like a playhouse in which you can play with your attention and become really good at spotlighting the many rooms in the house as well as discovering different thoughts. You can then decide what kind of thoughts you prefer to have.

(Lundgaard Bak, 2009: 40)

Storytelling is considered a very important part of our TiM workshops even though the TiM stories are very short stories. We are very careful about our storytelling performance and it is our experience that workshop participants are extremely attentive – there is always complete silence in the room and the impression is that people are clearly reflecting on the story in relation to their own thoughts and feelings. In nearly every workshop participants comment on their personal reflections of the stories and the TiM stories are also typically reflected upon again when we meet former participants maybe weeks or months later. Also the stories are often used by participants in their own practice (see examples later in the chapter, pp. 212–214). Thus we find that meta-narrative stories are very valuable mentalization metaphors.

The thinking brain and the alarm system

In the TiM project, the neuropsychology of mentalization is often demonstrated to parents and teachers by using Figure 11.3.

We note that in their everyday life, people have most certainly experienced being caught up in a thought or a feeling that is very hard to escape:

You have, for instance, heard a nice tune that keeps on playing inside your head – perhaps for hours . . . 'I just can't get that song off my mind.'

But we, both young and old people, also risk being trapped in much worse thoughts and feelings, such as anger or depression. The same is true when speaking of any type of *dependence* – and this results in partly loss of personal freedom and self-determination. The explanation is very often that the alarm system is over-sensitized.

Very unpleasant and dangerous situations (traumas, accidents, and assaults) increase the risk of over-sensitizing the feeling brain and the alarm system. Worst-case scenario is if the 'I' becomes totally 'out of your mind', which makes it difficult to find the way back to its own

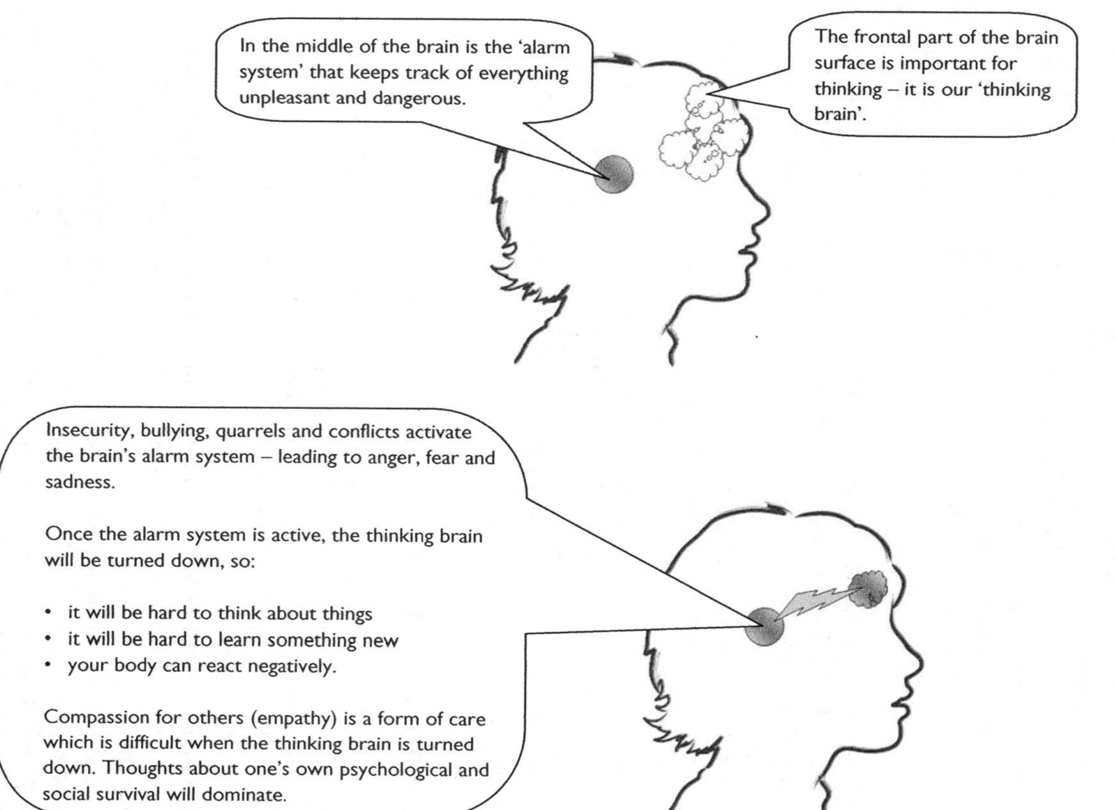

Figure 11.3 The thinking brain and the alarm system

> identity. In that case, the 'I' merges with the fear, and the person's life possibilities become limited.
>
> Random 'micro events' can, in unfortunate circumstances, also create permanent over-sensitivity in the alarm system (e.g. a horror film). The most frequent cause of imbalance in the alarm system is insecurity experienced in everyday life, e.g. 'micro bullying' in the family, in school, or at work.
>
> The thinking brain is put out of action when one becomes overwhelmed by feelings (for example, afraid, angry, or upset). This makes it very difficult to think sensibly – you simply react instinctively.
>
> (Lundgaard Bak, 2009: 22)

In the workshop and TiM material we then go on to discuss how the mind and brain can be trained by adequate challenges – as long as they are neither too large nor too small. Thus the thinking brain can learn to control the alarm centre so that the latter is not activated unintentionally, meaning that the alarm centre is stabilized and you become more resilient.[1] If the challenge is too large, the alarm centre takes over – the thinking brain turns down – and everything becomes difficult.

We go on to explain that humans and animals have the alarm system in common. However, the thinking brain is what makes us uniquely human, based on our highly developed frontal lobes. When we get annoyed and start arguing, we become more animal-like because we 'turn up the volume' of the alarm system and turn down the thinking brain. This is the case particularly if we feel personally affected by a critical or wounding remark. When we enter this 'animal-like' state of reacting, we really need to think sensibly in order to escape the trap.

Studies indicate that when the alarm system is 'switched on', its memory volume is turned up – while the thinking brain's memory volume is turned down (Levine, 1997; Rossi, 2002). It can therefore be difficult to remember details about what happened in a highly emotional situation after the event. This may explain why it is difficult for a child to relate to an unpleasant experience at a day-care centre or at school when he or she comes home. Once the child calms down, it is simply too difficult to remember details because the window into the feeling brain's memory is partly closed.

Explaining the brain's alarm centre to a child – and eventually letting the child draw/build his or her own alarm centre as he or she experiences it within – can be a good idea. Talking about situations where the child's alarm warning goes off – for better or for worse – and stimulating the child to think of ideas about what would be a good thing to do when this happens, can be very helpful. This provides the child with an understanding,

1 This is, of course, basically what is going on in cognitive behavioural training and, for that matter, in any well-organized learning process.

an overview, and courses of action regarding an important part of his or her inner system – that is psychoeducative mentalization training.

Many of the simple exercises in the TiM booklet and workshops can be of help to encourage adults and children to make better use of the 'thinking brain', provided that they are practised often, and thereby become 'an automatic reaction' when things are getting really difficult. For example, a simple, quiet question can often help a person who is at the mercy of his or her feelings: 'Tell me what is happening inside you right now.' When we describe how we feel inside, the thinking part of the brain is activated, and we are already on our way out of the animal-like behaviour.

In the TiM material, basic principles of cognitive behavioural training are also described as well as basic techniques of mental and body relaxation (for instance, breathing techniques), which of course are important factors to calm the alarm system and thereby create better conditions for mentalization in daily life.

The use of TiM techniques in different settings

Some examples of the various uses of the TiM techniques in school and day-care settings are given below:

A 15-year-old boy of normal intelligence frequently experiences severe anger complicated by severe aggressive behaviour even in minor teasing situations. He is motivated for change but is not sure how to achieve it. During a one-hour TiM conversation with a TiM trained teacher, he is told about the thinking brain and the alarm system. The TiM material is handed out to him. Three weeks later, he and his teacher report that he feels well and that there have been no episodes of violence. Two years later, he asks for a brush-up because he has had a minor relapse in connection with an educational problem. Otherwise, things go well for him.

A 16-year-old boy with a criminal record of violence has a series of conversations with a clinical psychologist. Their sessions simply centre on the question 'What are thoughts?' The boy has many reflections upon this question and expresses that he has never before been particular aware of what is going on inside himself. He finds this insight tremendously inspiring and helpful, and he restarts in a normal educational setting. During one of their conversations, the psychologist reads a small relaxing story from the TiM material, which is obviously comforting for the boy, and afterwards the boy says, 'I will go home and tell this story to my mother – she needs so much to relax.'

A mother reads the story from the TiM material about 'thought trains' to her 10-year-old son who has a school phobia. The boy reflects upon the story saying, 'Oh – I simply have to shift to another thought train inside myself.' His mother experiences that this insight is helpful to him in his process of going back to school.

A few weeks later, his ten years' older sister loses her boyfriend. Naturally she is sad, and then her little brother comes to her and says, 'Do you want me to read a story about a thought train for you?'

A 13-year-old girl has five conversations with a teacher knowledgeable in TiM techniques. The girl suffers from severe anxiety and shyness. Her family suffers from severe and complex problems. During their conversations, they make use of some of the TiM stories and transfer them into her life situation, her thoughts and feelings. Moreover, they visualize her thoughts and feelings by drawing 'thought bubbles'.

At the beginning of the fifth conversation, after entering the room, the girl sits down in the teacher's chair and says, 'Can you see what has happened?' Then she spontaneously does a half-an-hour session with the teacher as if the teacher was the client – including storytelling and creating appropriate challenges. Her way of expression and her body language have changed dramatically from the first to the fifth session.

A boy worries about walking around in the schoolyard because he tends to become extremely angry when teased by others. His teacher offers him information about the brain alarm system and how he can control the system. During several short sessions, he practises mental and body relaxation. Finally, they very carefully implement a cautious CBT-based plan with success, and he is gradually enabled to walk and play freely in the schoolyard. At the same time, teachers pay extra attention to the social climate in the schoolyard.

Together with their teacher, a tenth grade class has made a humorous and moving theatre play inspired by the TiM material where students play roles as professors, nerve cells, etc. In several tableaux they are illustrating central themes in teenage life, thoughts, and feelings – and the development and also vulnerability of the teenage brain.

The staff in a day-care centre has had a discussion about whether or not very early stimulation of mentalization is a possibility. They compare it with early language stimulation known to be important for proper language development. Trying it out, they write a small and very simple song for 2–3 year olds. The children obviously have fun with the song. Coincidentally, three months later, we meet with one of the mothers who tells us that her son, even several weeks after, is still playing with the song while pointing at his head and saying, 'I think, and I decide'.

In a class of students with special needs, including severe disruptive and violent behaviour, the staff has had a TiM training course. Despite their engagement, it has not been possible to conduct any meaningful TiM teaching with the students (probably because they are in high alarm and low mentalizing state of mind most of the time). However, the staff has found the concepts and knowledge about mentalization helpful in understanding the students' behaviour, and it has been helpful for them in order to stay calm in conflicts – thus helping them to create an evolved mentalizing environment. Within the first six months, they have succeeded in substantially reducing the frequency of conflict.

A two-hour TiM course has been held for a group of parents with severely obese children. It has raised a lot of different reflections in the group – upon hunger and craving, relations and attachment, and the teasing and bullying that their children are experiencing all too often. Immediately after the first session, a father asks the teacher in his daughter's class if he may visit the class and read the story of the House of Thoughts to the students. He wants them to know and realize more about the inner life of thoughts and feelings – to help them better understand his daughter.

Feasibility studies

The first feasibility study of the TiM project was conducted in autumn 2007. The leaders in the department for children and adolescents in Aarhus – a total of 656 head teachers, educational leaders, day-care staff, managers, etc. – were presented with the fundamental TiM concepts in a short lecture form. In a score for meaningfulness (range from 1–5), the average score was 4.8. In a later lecture series with a total of 348 employees participating, the average score was 4.4. The score was independent of the particular educator involved (a total of three educators gave the above lectures and courses). We have been very focused on the importance of high quality educational performance, and of course it is not easy to separate participant experience of educator performance from their experience of the relevance of mentalization as such. This is a basic condition in any educational process. The qualitative feedback from participants was used to expand and adjust the TiM material.

Between 2008 and 2010, a derived feasibility study was conducted based on the above-mentioned group of leaders who spontaneously demanded TiM presentations and courses for their staff. Presentations lasting between one and two hours were held on demand to more than 3500 employees in schools and day-care centres. Likewise, ten one-day TiM courses with 20 to 40 professional participants per day were held in 2009. Our interpretation of the overwhelming demand for this knowledge about mentalization was that the concepts and materials can be considered as meaningful for the staff working with children and adolescents.

In November 2009, a one-hour TiM evening lecture was held for approximately 500 parents in one of the schools in Aarhus (representing an unknown smaller number of families – because both mother and father may have joined the meeting). We announced that the TiM material could be downloaded from the school website the following morning. Within the first week, 230 copies of the TiM material were downloaded from the website.

During the feasibility study period, we have collected experiences and stories from professionals and parents who have started using the knowledge and inspiration from the TiM programme.

The most frequent comment from our participants after the lectures and courses is that they find the knowledge about mentalization relevant to their understanding of their own role in relationships with children, adolescents, and other adults in their daily life, especially in stressful situations and potential conflict situations. Here are some fairly representative statements from participants collected approximately one year after their participation in a TiM course:

> After the course, we made a presentation to our parents and it has been a topic of conversation in our teacher group ever since. I use it myself to influence thoughts that I give space to in my mind in stressful situations and periods. I often use 'the deep breath' technique in difficult conversations with parents or colleagues as a means to stay calm, be present and not let thoughts fly away. I think this is a lifelong learning process.

> We have learnt that we can become masters of our thoughts. We can ask inside ourselves why we think this way. Thoughts have real impact on the surroundings only when they are expressed – and not all thoughts need to be expressed. In our lives, we have to be present in the moment.

> TiM can hardly be distinguished from other instruments, but I want to emphasize that I have been seeking a greater focus on tasks in my daily life. I am probably more aware of what it takes from me and my personality to create peace around me. My focus in meetings with parents is sharpened, and I am clear and explicit in my expectations. In collaboration with my staff members, I have become more patient.

> I have used the TiM techniques in relation to myself and my family. You can choose to open or close the doors of the various emotions – and practise emotional control. The metaphor with the alarm brain and the thinking brain is very good and easy to remember.

Further evaluation studies

From the feasibility studies we conclude that the TiM programme raises sufficient interest among professionals and parents for it to be worth carrying out a more systematic evaluation of the approach. Two effect studies have been planned. The first one started in the winter of 2010, where we selected 15 schools, out of the 50 we support, to be our experimental group. The schools were selected to represent the social range of the schools in the city. The remaining 35 schools, which were carefully matched on a social ranking scale, represent the control group (except for two schools which are excluded from the study). The schools are located in low income multi-ethnic areas. Our strategy in these schools is to educate the staff so that they can use their knowledge about mentalization and the TiM tools in their daily work and contacts with students and parents. All parents and teachers from the experimental schools were invited to a two-hour TiM lecture and the TiM booklet and film were handed to the parents during the course. A follow-up will be carried out a year later and will be based on school attendance and academic results in relation to core questions from the WHO Health Behaviour in School-aged Children questionnaire (HBSC).[2]

The other study, which started in the spring of 2011, invited approximately 30 fourth grade classes (with a total of about 700 students) to a TiM course together with their parents. We use the same effect parameters as in the above-mentioned study and compare with another 120 fourth grade classes in the city.

In 2010, a 17-day postgraduate training course in mentalization was launched in Aarhus. The purpose is to educate 35 TiM supervisors – who will constitute a core group in the further development and research of the mentalization approach in the organization. They will be involved in the two evaluation studies mentioned above.

The study design is subject to the same limitations as other public health studies concerning, for example, control group matching and difficulties in blinding. The TiM project is already so well known in the organization that one cannot be sure that TiM activities are not taking place in the control group schools. We would therefore find it interesting to conduct studies with partners elsewhere in the country and internationally.

It is a limitation also that we have very limited knowledge about whether or not the effect parameters, primarily chosen because they are important general indicators of well-being and health, are sensitive parameters concerning the development of mentalizing communities, even though common sense may suggest a connection. As far as we know, no comparable studies exist, except for the Peaceful School projects referred to earlier (Twemlow *et al.*, Chapter 10), in which academic results have been used as effect parameters. If plausible effects can be traced on the chosen parameters, it is of course an interesting indication, but any findings will need to be treated with caution.

2 This is used in Aarhus to monitor mental health and health behaviour once every year in all 30,000 school students (since 2009).

Conclusion

Mentalization is clearly one of the most important factors behind mental health and behaviour. Hence, the development of mentalizing communities is of great interest both to the individual and to society. The preliminary results of the TiM project indicate that it may be possible and worthwhile to develop low-intensity, group-based programmes that are useful in making mentalizing ideas as widely available as possible among those caring for children, but further research is needed before firm conclusions can be made. The TiM project is among the first large-scale mentalization studies of this kind and we encourage researchers to develop and test further ideas in this field.

References

Fonagy, P., Gergely, G., Jurist, E., & Target, M. (2002). *Affect regulation, mentalization and the development of the self.* New York: Other Press.

Levine, P. (1997). *Waking the tiger. Healing trauma.* Berkeley, CA: North Atlantic Books.

Lundgaard Bak, P. (2009). *Thoughts in mind,* City of Aarhus.

Rossi, E. (2002). *The psychobiology of gene expression.* New York: Norton.

Index

AAI (Adult Attachment Interview) 14, 16
ADHD (attention deficit hyperactivity disorder) 71, 114
Adler, A. 198
Adolescent Levels of Emotional Awareness Scale (ALEAS) 60
adolescent mentalization-based integrative therapy (AMBIT) 163–85; basic stance 168–74; (clinical governance 172; individual keyworker relationship 169; intervening in multiple domains 171; respect for evidence 173–4; respect for local expertise 173; scaffolding existing relationships 172; taking responsibility for integration 171–2; well-connected team 171); challenges to implementation 167–8; complexity 164; core practices 175–6; (1. Thinking Together 176–80; 2. mentalizing the network 180–3; 3. manualizing the practice 173, 175, 183–4); current approaches 165–7; future developments 184–5; hard-to-reach young people 163–4; practice: (active planning 175; addressing network dis-integration 175, 182; mentalizing 174; supervisory structures 174; wiki manualization 175); Tower of Babel effect 164–5
adolescents: with borderline personality disorder 39–41; with depression 45; measurement of mentalization 59–62, 66–8; pseudomentalizing 44; psychopaths 44; with schizophrenia 38; *see also* adolescent mentalization-based integrative therapy (AMBIT); adolescents with chronic illness; mentalization-based treatment for adolescents (MBT-A); self-harm in young people
adolescents with chronic illness 147–61; biological measures evaluation 158–9; difficulties in mentalizing interpersonal stress 154–6; group modalities 151–2; mentalization-based group 156–8; mentalization-based therapy group model (MBTG-A) 152–4; paediatric end stage renal disease (ESRD) 148–50; pilot mentalization assessment 159–60; psychosocial impact 150–1
adopted children and their families 113–29; autobiographical continuity 117–18; challenges for adoptive parents 114–15; challenges for the adopted child 121–5; dissociation 123; impact of early experience on children 113–14; limit setting 119–20, 124–5; loss and dysregulation of emotions 125–8; MBT-F (mentalization-based treatment for families) 115–21; MBT in schools 121; play therapy 121–2, 126–8; projective identification 122–4; support for parents 117; therapeutic challenges 125–8; trauma 115, 121, 122–3, 127
Adult Attachment Interview (AAI) 14, 16
Adult Reflective Functioning Scale (ARFS) 64
affect and emotion: in adolescence 59, 136; affective mentalization 179;

affective understanding 56, 58–9, 62–4, 70; empathy 37, 44, 60; focus in MBT-P 90–1; instability in BPD 40–1; loss and dysregulation in adopted children 125–8; regulation 15, 20–2
Affect Knowledge Test (AKT) 56
Affect Task 62–4
agentive self: development 19–20
Ainsworth, M. D. S. et al. 14
ALEAS (Adolescent Levels of Emotional Awareness Scale) 60
alien self 134–5, 140–1
AMBIANCE (Atypical Maternal Behavior Instrument for Assessment and Classification) 16
AMBIT *see* adolescent mentalization-based integrative therapy
American Psychiatric Association 41
Anderson, B. et al. 151
Anna Freud Centre 7, 99
anxiety disorders 44–5, 59
ARFS (Adult Reflective Functioning Scale) 64
ASD (autistic spectrum disorders) 36–8
attachment: adopted children 113–14, 122; family discourse 16–17; impact of trauma 113–14; maltreatment 17–19; and mentalization 12, 13–19, 64–6; mentalizing and parenting 15–16; of patients with BPD 82–3; playfulness 17; security 14
attention deficit hyperactivity disorder (ADHD) 71, 114
attentional control 20–2
Atypical Maternal Behavior Instrument for Assessment and Classification (AMBIANCE) 16
authentic self 135
autistic spectrum disorders (ASD) 36–8
autobiographical continuity 117–18

Bales, D. et al. 80
Banerjee, R. 44–5
Baron-Cohen, S. et al. 36–8
Basic Empathy Scale (BES) 60
Bateman, A. 36, 88, 133, 134, 154
Beck, A. T. 44
Bergmann, T. 147, 148
Berkeley Puppet Interview (BPI) 56
biofeedback 19
Blair, R. J. et al. 44
borderline personality disorder (BPD) 12–13, 79; adolescents 39–41; core features 79–80; day-hospital MBT for adult BPD patients (MBT-DH) 79, 80; hyper-mentalizing 39–41; and impairments in mentalizing 79–81; importance of parental reflective functioning 80, 81–3; intensive outpatient MBT for adolescent BPD patients (MBT-A) 79; intensive outpatient MBT for BPD patients (MBT-IOP) 79, 80, 84, 85; and self-harm in young people 133; *see also* mentalization-based treatment for parents with BPD (MBT-P)
Bowlby, J. 13–14
BPI (Berkeley puppet interview) 56
brain: and attachment 15; mindreading 44; plasticity 59; *see also* 'Thoughts in Mind' project
British Child and Adolescent Mental Health Survey 41
Brock, J. 38, 39
Bronfman, E. et al. 16
bullying 43; *see also* Peaceful Schools experiment

CBT *see* cognitive behavioural therapy
CEMS (Children's Emotion Management Scale of Sadness and Anger) 59
Centre for Psychotherapy Viersprong 79
CGAS (Children's Global Assessment Scale) 109, 110
Child and Adolescent Mental Health Services (CAMHS) 64, 113, 135, 140, 181
Child and Adolescent Social Perception Scale (CASPS) 60
Child Attachment Interview (CAI) 64
Child Reflective Functioning Scale (CRFS) 64–6
children: with anxiety disorders 44–5, 59; autistic children 36–8; bullies 43; with depression 26, 45, 71; externalizing behaviour problems 41–3; interpersonal difficulties 41; self *vs.* other focus 69–70; *see also* adopted children and their families; infants; preschoolers and toddlers; primary-school-age children

Children's Emotion Management Scale of Sadness and Anger (CEMS) 59
Children's Global Assessment Scale (CGAS) 109, 110
Child's Eye Task 42, 43
circular questioning 100
Clark, D. A. 44
Clay, D. L. et al. 150
Cleckley, H. 44
clinic-based interventions *see* adopted children and their families; mentalization-based treatment for families (MBT-F); mentalization-based treatment for parents with BPD (MBT-P); self-harm in young people
cognitive behavioural therapy (CBT) 58, 100, 166, 171, 179, 212
cognitive modularist view 36
Colombo style curiosity 108–9
community-based interventions *see* adolescent mentalization-based integrative therapy (AMBIT); adolescents with chronic illness; Peaceful Schools experiment; 'Thoughts in Mind' project (TiM)
Complexity of Representations subscale 61
conduct disorder 41, 114
core self 133
CRFS (Child Reflective Functioning Scale) 64–6
Crick, N. R. 43
culture 72, 150, 158
Cunningham, J. N. et al. 59
curiosity 25, 26, 43, 88–9, 100, 108–9, 116, 203

Daleiden, E. L. 44
day-hospital MBT for adult BPD patients (MBT-DH) 79, 80
De Shazer, S. 100
Dennett, D. 54, 190
depression: in adolescents 45; in adults 45; in children 26, 45, 71; in parents 25
dissociation in adopted children 123
distorted mentalizing 36, 41–3, 58
Dodge, K. A. et al. 41
Dunn, J. et al. 56
Dziobek, I. et al. 35, 60

Ecole Psychosomatique de Paris 12
Ekman, P. et al. 62
emotion *see* affect and emotion
empathy 37, 44, 60
Ensink, K. et al. 66
ESRD (paediatric end stage renal disease) 148–50
evaluation 6–7; adolescents with chronic illness 158–60; AMBIT programme 184; of MBT-F 109–10; in MBT-P 85–6; 'Thoughts in Mind' project (TiM) 215–16
existential susceptibility 122
Experience of Service Questionnaire (ESQ) 110
explicit mentalizing group training 87–8
externalizing behaviour problems 41–3

false belief tasks 16, 17, 21, 36–7, 41, 56, 59, 60, 61
families: enmeshed families 26; mentalizing in 23–7; *see also* adopted children and their families; mentalization-based treatment for families (MBT-F)
family discourse 16–17
family support services 99
Faux Pas Test 57
Flavell, J. H. et al. 57
Fonagy, P. et al. 1, 12, 79–80, 88, 98, 102, 133, 134, 147, 154
foster parents *see* parents
Fowler, D. et al. 108
Freud, A. 147, 148
Frith, U. et al. 44

Garralda, M. E. et al. 151
Gergely, G. et al. 19, 55
Goodyer, I. 45
Grotpeter, J. K. 43
group work: explicit mentalizing group training for parents 87–8; mentalization-based therapy group model (MBTG-A) 152–4; *see also* adolescents with chronic illness

Happé's Strange Stories (HSS) 56–7
hard-to-reach young people *see* adolescent mentalization-based integrative therapy (AMBIT)
Harris, P. L. 59
Hartmann, D. P. 71

Health Behaviour in School-aged Children questionnaire (HBSC) 216
Health of the Nation Outcome Scales for Children and Adolescents (HoNOSCA) 109, 110
Higgitt, A. 12
Hill, J. et al. 16–17
Hirsch, N. 60
Hofer, M. A. 15
horizontal decolage 46
hospital settings *see* adolescents with chronic illness
HSS (Happé's Strange Stories) 56–7
hyper-mentalizing 25, 36; in borderline personality disorder 39–41; in schizophrenia 38–9
hypothalamic-pituitary-adrenal (HPA) axis 40

identification with the aggressor 18
infants: measurement of mentalization 55; *see also* mentalization-based treatment for parents with BPD (MBT-P)
insightfulness 15
intensive outpatient MBT for adolescent BPD patients (MBT-A) 79
intensive outpatient MBT for BPD patients (MBT-IOP) 79, 80, 84, 85
internal working models (IWMs) 14
interpersonal difficulties 41

Jemerin, J. 115
joining 100

Kettle, J. L. et al. 45
Klein, M. 125
Koren-Karie, N. 15–16
Kusche, C. A. et al. 58
Kusche's Affective Interview (KAI-R) 58
Kyte, Z. 45

Langdon, R. 38, 39
language abilities 72
learning disabilities 71, 114
Lee, L. et al. 45
Leslie, A. M. 12
Linehan, M. M. 40
Lundgaard Bak, P. 203–4, 205, 206–9, 211

Main, M. 16–17
Malberg, N. T. et al. 152
maltreatment of children 17–19
manipulativeness 18
manualization of MBT: AMBIT programme 173, 175, 183–4; MBT-F 101; wiki manualization 175
MAPI (Millon Adolescent Personality Interview) 156
MASC (Movie for the Assessment of Social Cognition) 35–6, 60
maternal mind-mindedness (MMM) 15, 81–3
MBT (mentalization-based treatment) 1–2
MBT-A *see* mentalization-based treatment for adolescents
MBT-DH (day-hospital MBT for adult BPD patients) 79, 80
MBT-F *see* mentalization-based treatment for families
MBT in schools 121
MBT-IOP *see* intensive outpatient MBT for BPD patients
MBT-P *see* mentalization-based treatment for parents with BPD
MBTG-A (mentalization-based therapy group model) 152–4
MDFT (multidimensional family therapy) 166–7
measurement of mentalization 54–73; in adolescents 59–62, 66–8; affective understanding 62–4, 70; in attachment relationships 64–6; indirect manifestation 71; influences on task performance 71–2; integrating cognitive and affective aspects 61–8; mentalization capacities 68–9; pleasant or unpleasant states of mind 70; in preschoolers and toddlers 55–6, 69; in primary-school-age children 56–9, 61–6; in real life 70–1; role of context 70; self-report measures 60; self *vs.* other focus 69–70; use in outcome research 72
Meins, E. et al. 15–16
mental states 70
mentalization: affective mentalization 179; and attachment 12, 13–19, 64–6; capacities 68–9; concept 1, 11;

definitional overlap 55; emergence in children 12–13; loss of mentalizing 23–7; misuse of 27; origins of the concept 12–13; *see also* measurement of mentalization
mentalization-based therapy group model (MBTG-A) 152–4
mentalization-based treatment (MBT) 1–2; *see also* day-hospital MBT for adult BPD patients (MBT-DH); intensive outpatient MBT for BPD patients (MBT-IOP); MBT in schools; mentalization-based therapy group model (MBTG-A); mentalization-based treatment for adolescents (MBT-A); mentalization-based treatment for families (MBT-F); mentalization-based treatment for parents with BPD (MBT-P)
mentalization-based treatment for adolescents (MBT-A) 79, 135–40; aim and emphasis 135–6; assessment phase 136–7; initial treatment phase 137; middle phase 137–8; final phase 138; emotional dysregulation 136; formulation meeting 137; key elements 136; psychoeducation meeting 137
mentalization-based treatment for families (MBT-F) 79, 98–111; aims 100; introductory session 101–3; adopted children and their families 115–21; family support services 99; holding the balance 103–7; initial evaluation 109–10; manualization 101; MBT-F loop 107–9; therapeutic aspects 100; therapeutic stance 104–5
mentalization-based treatment for parents with BPD (MBT-P) 79–94; challenge and praise 92–3; core features of BPD 79–80; crisis plan 86; explicit mentalizing group training 87–8; focus of programme 83–4; focus on affect 90–1; focus on current mental states 90; focus on parental strengths 92; individual parent–infant psychotherapy 86–7; mentalizing in the current parent–infant relationship 93; modelling parental reflectiveness 91–2; parental reflective functioning (PRF) 81–3, 84, 86–7; parents: definition 83; pedagogical stance 89–90; programme ingredients 84–5; therapeutic stance 88–9; treatment planning 85–6; video-feedback interventions 86–7, 91
mentalization capacities 68–9
mentalizing: cognitive modularist view 36; distorted mentalizing 36, 41–3, 58; explicit mentalizing group training 87–8; in families 23–7; hyper-mentalizing 25, 36, 38–41; impairments in BPD 79–81; loss of mentalizing 23–7; no mentalizing 36; and parenting 15–16; pseudomentalizing 26, 36, 43–4; and theory of mind (ToM) 36, 43, 45; under-mentalizing 36, 37–8
Mentalizing Stories for Adolescents (MSA) 66–8
Millon Adolescent Personality Interview (MAPI) 156
mind-blindness 37
mindfulness 45
Minding the Baby programme 82, 86
mindreading 43
Minuchin, S. 100
mirroring 19, 20, 89, 115, 122, 127–8, 133
MMM (maternal mind-mindedness) 15, 81–3
Moran, G. 147
Movie for the Assessment of Social Cognition (MASC) 35–6, 60
MSA (Mentalizing Stories for Adolescents) 66–8
multidimensional family therapy (MDFT) 166–7
multisystemic therapy (MST) 166

Nesse, R. M. 39
no mentalizing 36

object relations theory 125–6
O'Connor, T. 60
Ogden, T. 198
Oppenheim, D. 15–16
oppositional behaviour 18
oppositional defiant disorder 41
Oprell, D. 122
outcome measures 72

outpatient therapy *see* intensive outpatient MBT for BPD patients (MBT-IOP); mentalization-based treatment for adolescents (MBT-A)

paediatric end stage renal disease (ESRD) 148–50
parental reflective functioning (PRF) 79; in borderline personality disorder 80, 81–3; in MBT-P programme 81–3, 84, 86–7, 91–2
parents: definition 83; with depression 25; and mentalizing 15–16; mentalizing in families 23–7; with schizophrenia 25; *see also* adopted children and their families; families; mentalization-based treatment for parents with BPD (MBT-P)
Parents First programme 82
Patterson, C. C. 16
pause and review 104–5
Peaceful Schools experiment 187–200; a problem child 187–9; mentalization perspective 189–93; a mentalizing social system 195–9; (classroom management (discipline plan) 196–7; gentle warrior physical education programmes 198; peer and adult mentorship 197–8; positive climate campaigns 196; reflection time 198–9); results of the projects 199–200; social systems-power dynamics perspective 193–5
perspective taking 44
Piaget, J. 46
Pivnick, B. A. 125, 129
Plante, W. A. et al. 152
play therapy 121–2, 126–8
playfulness 17, 98, 110
Pons, F. 59
preschoolers and toddlers: influences on task performance 71; measurement of mentalization 55–6, 69; theory of mind 56
pretend mode 21, 23, 98, 106, 127
PRF *see* parental reflective functioning
primary-school-age children: affective understanding 56, 58–9, 62–4, 70; attachment relationships 64–6; distorted mentalizing 41–3, 58; externalizing behaviour problems 41–3; measurement of mentalization 56–9, 61–6; misperception of thoughts/feelings of others 57–8; theory of mind 22, 56
projective identification 18, 106; in adopted children 122–4
pseudomentalizing 26, 36, 43–4
psychic equivalence 21, 23, 125, 126
psychodynamic practice/perspective 58, 100, 147, 160
psychopaths 44

Quinodoz, D. 125

randomized controlled trials (RCT): in gang membership 184; in multi-dimensional family therapy 167; Peaceful Schools Project 196, 199; in self-harm in young people 5, 131
Reading the Mind in the Eyes Test (RMET) 57, 58
reflective function (RF) 15, 55, 65
Reflective Functioning Questionnaire–Adolescent (RFQ-A) 60
Richell, R. A. et al. 42
roletaking 44

Sandler, J. 100
schizophrenia 25, 38–9
school-based interventions; *see* MBT in schools; Peaceful Schools experiment; 'Thoughts in Mind' project
SCORS (Social Cognition and Object Relation Scale) 61
SDQ (Strengths and Difficulties Questionnaire) 109–10
seeing-leads-to-knowing tests 37
self: alien self 134–5, 140–1; authentic self 135; core self 133; development of the agentive self 19–20; *vs.* other focus 69–70
self-harm in young people 131–42; alien self 134–5, 140–1; and borderline personality disorder (BPD) 133; co-morbidity 132–3; incidence 132; intention 132–3; MBT-A (mentalization-based treatment for adolescents) 135–40; mentalization-based framework 133–5
self-report measures 60
Selvini Palazzoli, M. et al. 100

sensory disabilities 71
Sharp, C. et al. 39, 42, 58
Shmueli-Goetz, Y. et al. 64–5
Siegal, M. 16
Slade, A. et al. 15, 16
SMART (short-term mentalizing and relational therapy) 99n
social biofeedback 19
social cognition 19–20, 41, 44, 45, 60
Social Cognition and Object Relation Scale (SCORS) 61
social information processing theory 44–5
social intelligence 14–15
Social Situations Task 57
Soliday, E. et al. 150
Sroufe, L. A. 14–15
START criteria 180
Steele, M. et al. 128
Strange Situation 14
Strengths and Difficulties Questionnaire (SDQ) 109–10
stress 24, 40
subjectivity before mentalization 22–3
Sutton, J. et al. 43
systemic practice and perspective 25–6, 100, 102, 156, 165–6, 172

Target, M. et al. 12, 98
taxonomy 35–6
teachers *see* MBT in schools; Peaceful Schools experiment; 'Thoughts in Mind' project
teleological mode 23
Test of Emotional Comprehension (TEC) 59
Thematic Apperception Test (TAT) 61
theory of mind (ToM): advanced ToM measures 59; cognitive-linguistic aspects 56–7; Faux Pas Test 57; introspection skills 57; and mentalizing 36, 43, 45; in preschool age children 56; in primary-school-age children 22, 56; Reading the Mind in the Eyes Test (RMET) 57, 58; Social Situations Task 57; Test of Emotional Comprehension (TEC) 59; third-order tasks 56–7
Thinking Together 176–80; 1. marking the task 177–8; 2. stating the case 178–9; 3. mentalizing the moment 179; 4. returning to purpose 179–80
'Thoughts in Mind' project (TiM) 202–17; basic concepts 203–9; feasibility studies 214–15; further evaluation studies 215–16; project development 202–3; story of the House of Thoughts 208–9; the thinking brain and the alarm system 209–12; use of techniques in different settings 212–14
TiddlySpace 184
TiddlyWiki 101, 184
TiM *see* 'Thoughts in Mind' project
toddlers *see* preschoolers and toddlers
ToM *see* theory of mind
Tower of Babel effect 164–5
trauma: in adopted children 115, 121, 122–3, 127; effect on capacity to 'play' 98; effects on HPA axis 40; impact on attachment 113–14; *see also* adolescents with chronic illness
trust behaviour 42–3

under-mentalizing 36, 37–8
Understanding Social Causality subscale 61

Van den Dries, L. 114
Vasey, M. W. 44
video-feedback interventions 86–7, 91
Viersprong Institute for Studies on Personality Disorders (VISPD) 79

Watling, D. 44–5
Watson, J. 19
Wimmer, H. et al. 37n
Winnicott, D. W. 20, 103, 125

Zeman, J. 69